Traumatic Experiences and Dyslexia

Beiträge zur Pädagogischen und
Rehabilitationspsychologie

Studies in Educational and
Rehabilitation Psychology

Herausgegeben von / Edited by Evelin Witruk

Bd./Vol. 8

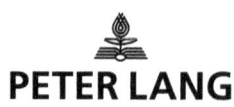

Evelin Witruk / Dian Sari Utami (eds.)

# Traumatic Experiences and Dyslexia

PETER LANG

**Bibliographic Information published by the Deutsche Nationalbibliothek**
The Deutsche Nationalbibliothek lists this publication in the Deutsche
Nationalbibliografie; detailed bibliographic data is available on the Internet
at http://dnb.d-nb.de.

**Library of Congress Cataloging-in-Publication Data**
A CIP catalog record for this book has been applied for at the Library of
Congress.

ISSN 1865-083X
ISBN 978-3-631-73191-8 (Print)
E-ISBN 978-3-631-79598-9 (E-Book)
E-ISBN 978-3-631-79599-6 (E-PDF)
E-ISBN 978-3-631-79600-9 (MOBI)
DOI 10.3726/b15891

© Peter Lang GmbH
Internationaler Verlag der Wissenschaften
Berlin 2019
All rights reserved.
PL Academic Research is an imprint of Peter Lang GmbH.

Peter Lang – Berlin · Bern · Bruxelles · New York ·
Oxford · Warszawa · Wien

All parts of this publication are protected by copyright. Any
utilisation outside the strict limits of the copyright law, without
the permission of the publisher, is forbidden and liable to
prosecution. This applies in particular to reproductions,
translations, microfilming, and storage and processing in
electronic retrieval systems.

This publication has been peer reviewed.

www.peterlang.com

# Contents

List of Contributors .................................................................................. 9

Preface ..................................................................................................... 11

## Chapter 1 Traumatic Experiences

*Konrad Reschke, Anar Bikadamova, & Gulzat Sarbassova*
Psychological First Aid ............................................................................ 19

*Hamidreza Khankeh & Elham Sepahvand*
Concept Analysis of Bystander Effect in Road Traffic Injuries: A
Hybrid Model ........................................................................................... 25

*Juliet Roudini, Hamidreza Khankeh, Evelin Witruk, Abbas Ebadi, Konrad Reschke, & Marcus Stueck*
Dimensions of Community Mental Health Preparedness of Disasters
in Iran ....................................................................................................... 33

*Johanna Sophie von Lieres*
Mental Well-Being and Protective Factors in Vulnerable
Groups: Victims of the 2004 Tsunami in Kerala, South India, and
Disadvantaged Rural Populations in North India ................................. 45

*Asanka Bulathwatta and Evelin Witruk*
Trauma and Coping Styles among University Students in Sri Lanka
and Germany: Role of Emotional Intelligence and Resilience ............ 59

*Nadia Hanum*
Trauma after Accident: Case Study of Traffic Accident Survivors with
Spinal Cord Injury in Indonesia ............................................................. 65

## Chapter 2  Stress Experiences

*Marcus Stueck, Hans-Ullrich Balzer, Sebastian Mueller,
Dian Sari Utami, & Ulrich Sack*
Das mobile Gesundheitslabor: Ein Bestandteil des
Gesundheitswürfels zur Psychischen Gefährdungs- und
Ressourcenbeurteilung im Rahmen des Biozentrisch-betrieblichen
Gesundheitsmanagements ............................................................................ 73

*Marcus Stueck*
Der Gesundheitswürfel: Ein Instrument zur Psychischen
Gefährdungs- und Ressourcenbeurteilung im Rahmen des
Biozentrischen und Betrieblichen Gesundheitsmanagements in
Unternehmen und Institutionen ................................................................. 91

*I. P. R. Chathuranga, Buddhiphraba D. D. Pathirana, & Marcus Stueck*
Cultural Adaptation of Biodanza to Manage Stress within Sri Lankan
Youth and Adolescence ............................................................................... 107

*Edgar Galindo*
Teaching Academic, Social and Independence Skills to Slum Children ...... 115

*Dian Sari Utami & Evelin Witruk*
Parenting Stressors and Positive Coping among Indonesian Parents
with a Deaf or Hard-of-Hearing Schoolchild ............................................. 135

*Gunendra R. K. Dissanayake*
Most Frequent and Distressing Forms of Intimate Partner
Psychological Abuse among Women in Sri Lankan Context .................... 143

*Emi Zulaifah, Hazhira Qudsyi, Rumiani, & Sri Wahyuningsih*
Strategies for Controlling Internet Usage in Dual-Earner Families ........... 151

*Bagus Riyono & Annisa Rizkiayu Leofianti*
The Role of Social Support to Cope with Work-Family Conflict .............. 159

## Chapter 3  Dyslexia

*Evelin Witruk*
Dyslexia – Does It Still Exist? ..................................................................... 169

*Mahnaz Akhavan Tafti*
Dyslexia: Disabled or Differently Abled .............................................................. 175

*Samudra Senarath*
Anxiety and Self-Esteem among Children with Dyslexia in Sri Lanka ........ 189

*Enoka Randeniya*
Comprehensive Reading Difficulties on Sinhala Language of Dyslexic
Students in Sri Lanka .............................................................................................. 197

*Francisca Serrano*
The Emotional Profile in Children with Dyslexia and Learning
Disabilities ................................................................................................................. 205

*Isabel Leite & Tânia Fernandes*
A Dark Consequence of Developmental Dyslexia: Discrimination of
Mirror Images is not Automatized ....................................................................... 215

*Adil Ishag*
The Impact of Diglossia on Arabic Reading Comprehension ......................... 227

*Raziq Ouafa*
Die Bedeutsamkeit des Phänomens Legasthenie in Marokko ......................... 233

*Khaled Youssef Alammar*
A Study of Dyslexia among Fourth Class Pupils in Rural Daraa
according to Some Variables .................................................................................. 239

# List of Contributors

**Mahnaz Akhavan Tafti**
Alzahra University, Iran

**Khaled Youssef Alammar**
Damascus University, Syria

**Hans-Ullrich Balzer**
Humboldt-Universität Berlin, Germany

**Anar Bikadamova**
Al-Farabi Kazakh National University, Almaty, Kazakhstan

**Asanka Bulathwatta**
University of Peradeniya, Sri Lanka

**I. P. R. Chathuranga**
University of Peradeniya, Sri Lanka

**Gunendra R. K. Dissanayake**
University of Peradeniya, Sri Lanka

**Abbas Ebadi**
University of Baqiyatallah University of Medical Sciences, Iran

**Tânia Fernandes**
University of Lisboa, Portugal

**Edgar Galindo**
University of Evora, Portugal

**Nadia Hanum**
University of Leipzig, Germany

**Adil Ishag**
International University of Africa, Sudan

**Hamidreza Khankeh**
University of Social Welfare and Rehabilitation Sciences, Iran

**Isabel Leite**
University of Évora, Portugal

**Annisa Rizkiayu Leofianti**
Universitas Gadjah Mada, Indonesia

**Johanna Sophie von Lieres**
Center for Women's Empowerment and Gender Equality Amrita Vishwa Vidyapeetham Amritapuri, India

**Sebastian Mueller**
International Research Academy-BIONET, Germany

**Raziq Ouafa**
Université Hassan II, Morocco

**Buddhiphraba D. D. Pathirana**
University of Peradeniya, Sri Lanka

**Hazhira Qudsyi**
Islamic University of Indonesia, Indonesia

**Enoka Randeniya**
University of Colombo, Sri Lanka

**Konrad Reschke**
University of Leipzig, Germany

**Bagus Riyono**
Universitas Gadjah Mada, Indonesia

**Juliet Roudini**
University of Leipzig, Germany

**Rumiani**
Islamic University of Indonesia, Indonesia

**Ulrich Sack**
Universität Leipzig, Germany

**Gulzat Sarbassova**
Al-Farabi Kazakh National University, Almaty, Kazakhstan

**Samudra Senarath**
University of Colombo, Sri Lanka

**Elham Sepahvand**
University of Social Welfare and Rehabilitation of Sciences, Iran

**Francisca Serrano**
University of Granada, Spain

**Marcus Stueck**
DPFA Academy for Work and Health, Germany
DPFA-Akademie für Arbeitsgesundheit
International Research
Academy – BIONET

**Dian Sari Utami**
Institute of Psychology, University of Leipzig, Germany
Islamic University of Indonesia, Indonesia

**Sri Wahyuningsih**
Islamic University of Indonesia, Indonesia

**Evelin Witruk**
Institute of Psychology, University of Leipzig, Germany

**Emi Zulaifah**
Islamic University of Indonesia, Indonesia

# Preface

This book presents as the eight bands in the series of "Contributions to Educational and Rehabilitation Psychology". It contains selected contributions from the international conference "Dyslexia and Traumatic Experiences" organized by the team members of the Department of Educational and Rehabilitation Psychology of the Institute of Psychology at the University of Leipzig. It took place on 22nd and 23rd of September 2017 in the University of Leipzig, Leipzig, Germany. Fifty-one of international participants came from Indonesia, Sri Lanka, India, Morocco, Sudan, South Korea, Iran, Portugal, Spain, and Germany. In the same time, it was an interdisciplinary one because scientists from Psychology, Education, and Special Education attended this event. The conference had offered a platform for integrating basic and applied sciences, especially in the topic of dyslexia, trauma, and stress experiences. It brought together Cognitive, Educational, Clinical Psychologists, and Neuropsychological specialists. Particular participants in the international conference were scientists from Sri Lanka and Sudan which were sponsored by the Research Academy of the University of Leipzig regarding their research about dyslexic children and traumatic experiences.

The purpose of this book is to strive towards fostering a scientific exchange that promotes the emergence of synergy effects and real progress in the understanding of cross-cultural aspects and to present fundamental approaches and applied for work in the special issues of trauma, stress experiences, and dyslexia as the main foci in the international conference.

The book is structured in **three chapters**, in which the following topics are introduced:

**Chapter 1** includes articles regarding **Traumatic Experiences**. The first chapter is focused on the topic of traumatic experiences in Germany, Kazhastan, Iran, India, Sri Lanka, and Indonesia. Konrad Reschke from the University of Leipzig together with Anar Bikadamova, and Gulzat Sarbassova from the Al-Farabi Kazakh National University, Almaty in Kazakhstan give an overview of Psychological First Aid. Hamidreza Khankeh and Elham Sepahvand from the University of Social Welfare and Rehabilitation of Sciences in Iran discuss the phenomenon of the Bystander effect in road traffic injuries and apply the hybrid model. The next article is from Juliet Roudini, Hamidreza Khankeh, Evelin Witruk, Abbas Ebadi, Konrad Reschke, and Marcus Stueck from the University of Leipzig, Germany, the University of Social Welfare and Rehabilitation Sciences in Iran, the University of Baqiyatallah University of Medical Sciences in Iran, and the DPFA Academy for Work and Health in Germany. They give an overview of the dimensions of community mental health preparedness of the disasters in Iran.

Further, Johanna Sophie von Lieres from the Center for Women's Empowerment and Gender Equality Amrita Vishwa Vidyapeetham Amritapuri in India reports about well-being and protective factors in vulnerable groups in India. She selected for the study victims of the 2004 Tsunami in Kerala in South India, and disadvantaged rural populations in North India. Asanka Bulathwatta and Evelin Witruk from the University of Peradeniya, Sri Lanka and the University of Leipzig, Germany report on trauma and coping styles among university students in Sri Lanka and Germany and discuss the role of emotional intelligence and resilience. As the last author in this chapter, Nadia Hanum from the University of Leipzig in Germany which focuses on the trauma after the accident and reports a case study of traffic accident survivors with spinal cord injury in Indonesia.

**Chapter 2** involves contributions regarding **Stress Experiences.** Stress experiences in different life situations can impact the personality and can lead to serious health problems within individual and family. It is explained by scientists from Germany, Sri Lanka, Portugal, and Indonesia. The first article is from Marcus Stueck, Hans-Ulrich Balzer, Sebastian Mueller, Dian Sari Utami, and Ulrich Sack from the DPFA Academy of Work and Health, Humboldt-University Berlin, Islamic University of Indonesia, and the University of Leipzig in Germany. They report about the mobile health labour as a method for measurement of risks and resources among people. Also, Marcus Stueck from the DPFA Academy of Work and Health continues his report about the health cube, which allows the measurement of risks and resources on six levels. The third article is from I. P. R. Chathuranga, Budhiphraba D. D. Pathirana and Marcus Stueck from the University of Peradeniya, Sri Lanka and DPFA Academy of Work and Health, Germany. They report about the cultural adaptation of biodanza to manage stress within Sri Lankan youth and adolescence.

Further, Edgar Galindo from the University of Evora in Portugal reports on teaching academic, social and independence skills to slum children. The next article is from Dian Sari Utami and Evelin Witruk from the Islamic University of Indonesia and the University of Leipzig in Germany report about parenting stressors and positive coping among Indonesian parents with a deaf or hard-of-hearing schoolchild. Also, Gunendra R. K. Dissanayake discusses the most frequent and distressing forms of the intimate partner psychological abuse among women in the Sri Lankan context.

Furthermore, some researchers from Indonesia, Emi Zulaifah, Hazhira Qudsyi, Rumiani, and Sri Wahyuningsih from the Islamic University of Indonesia discuss the strategies for controlling internet usage in dual-earner families. Also, Bagus Riyono and Annisa Rizkiayu Leofianti from the University of Gadjah Mada, Indonesia give an overview of the role of social support to cope with the work-family conflict.

**Chapter 3** is focused on **Dyslexia.** It is the last chapter and discusses the topic of reasons and consequences of dyslexia in Germany, Iran, Sri Lanka, Spain, Portugal, Morocco, and Syria. Evelin Witruk from the University of Leipzig, Germany gives an overview of the methods of assessment and intervention and explains a new perspective of dyslexia on an old phenomenon and the giftedness of dyslexics. The second article from Mahnaz Akhavan Tafti from Alzahra University in Teheran, Iran explains about talents and giftedness among dyslexic children and adults. The discussion of children with dyslexia has also been addressed in the next article by Samudra Senarath from the University of Colombo, Sri Lanka about secondary symptoms and special topics about anxiety and self-esteem as mechanism among dyslexic children. Also, comprehensive reading difficulties on the Sinhala language of dyslexic students in Sri Lanka will be explained by Enoka Randeniya from the University of Colombo.

Further, Francisca Serrano from the University of Granada in Spain measured the emotional profile in children with dyslexia and learning disabilities. She could show higher values in anxiety, and lower values in self-concept and self-esteem in dyslexic children. A dark consequence of developmental dyslexia is explained in the next part by Isabel Leite and Tânia Fernandes from the University of Évora and the University of Lisboa in Portugal. In this article, they could show that the discrimination of mirror images is not automatised.

Furthermore, three articles from the Arabic speaking area are integrated into this chapter. Adil Ishag from the International University of Africa in Sudan discusses the impact of Diglossia on Arabic reading comprehension, and he explains the problems of the dyslexic children. Raziq Ouafa from the Université Hassan II, Morocco focuses on the interview results among teachers from Casablanca about the relevance of the phenomenon of dyslexia in Morocco. The last but not least is the study from Khaled Youssef Alammar from Damascus University in Syria that gives interesting results about dyslexia among fourth class pupils in rural Daraa.

All of the chapters above are work reports from many researchers across countries that are integrated mostly in the presentations on the workshop "Dyslexia and Traumatic Experiences". Therefore, those works and scientists are keeping to interact and collaborate with others.

Evelin Witruk and Dian Sari Utami

# Acknowledgement

The participants of the workshop, the authors of the book articles, and as well as the editors were very grateful for the sponsorship of the Research Academy of the University of Leipzig and from the Islamic University of Indonesia for the scientists from Sri Lanka, Sudan and Indonesia.

Evelin Witruk & Dian Sari Utami
Leipzig, February 2019

# Chapter 1  Traumatic Experiences

Konrad Reschke, Anar Bikadamova, & Gulzat Sarbassova

# Psychological First Aid

**Abstract:** Some aspects, actions and strategies of psychological first aid will be discussed in the first part. Main part will focus on and draw attention to learning possibilities and training in psychological first aid. The German-speaking authors Lasogga and Gasch (2011), who proposed a model, will be outlined.

**Keywords:** psychological first aid, learning procedures

## 1 What is Psychological First Aid (PFA)?

In this first part, we will describe what psychological first aid is. In the context of a disaster, psychologists can deliver a special kind of help, psychological first aid. It is also possible by all other urgency forces if they are trained and able and willing to do this social and psychological service additionally in the moments of early help which will be given.

Psychological First Aid is an evidence-formed modular approach to help in the immediate aftermath of disaster, emergency or terrorism. It is designed to reduce initial distress and to prevent post-traumatic stress disorder, adjustment disorder and acute stress disorder (PTSD, AD and ASD). PFA serves to foster short- and long-term adaptive functioning and coping of the victims and overcome helplessness of the victims. PFA is the practice of recognising and responding to people who need help because they are feeling stress, resulting from the disaster situations within which they find themselves.

Knowing how to provide Psychological First Aid can help you to:

a) Create a compassionate environment for disaster survivors and workers.
b) Assess what a person might need at a particular time.
c) Provide immediate support to those in stressful situations.
d) Help others cope in the face of stressful events.
e) Prevention of PTSD and acute stress disorders, and adjustment disorder

Who can deliver PFA? Designed for delivery by mental health workers and other disaster response workers within a wide variety of response units:

a) First responder teams
b) Health care providers of different professions
c) School crisis response teams,
d) Crisis intervention teams,
e) Particular NGO's and helping organizations (like Red Cross, etc.)

The Basic objectives of PFA are: 1) Establish a human connection in a non-intrusive, compassionate manner; 2) Enhance immediate and ongoing safety and provide physical and emotional comfort; 3) Calm and orient emotionally overwhelmed or distraught survivors or helpers; and 4) Offer practical assistance and information to address immediate needs/concerns.

The need for PFA comes from the following facts 1) that the probability of disaster is always given and 2) there is an everyday disaster risk. Thus, 3) we have to understand it because there are disaster-prone regions with higher risks.

Disasters may create significant impairment in 40–50% of those exposed Norris, Friedman, & Watson, 2002). Hence, disaster preparedness is needed. The PFA is included in disaster resilience strategy and disaster preparedness. Further, in this chapter, we will outline the most critical actions (core actions) and strategy of PFA.

## 2 Core Actions and Strategies of PFA

The core actions and strategies of PFA includes all that can provide early assistance within days or weeks following a disaster or critical event in disasters format. The psychological post-disaster help act seldom in the first row of disaster help. However, when the disaster strikes, survivors may need more than just physical assistance. They may also require Psychological First Aid for disaster-caused trauma and stress. Severe cases will require the support of a mental health professional.

For many, however, the best medicine you can provide is often given by empathic caregivers. Some Easy Rules can help to help in this situation. Lasogga and Gasch (2011) proposed the "4S" rule in the followings:

1. Say who you are
2. Say, that you are here
3. Say, that you will stay
4. Say, what you do

Whereas in the STOP model of Red Cross, it will give another frame, how people must be helped in the case of disaster. These needs are:

1. S - Safety
2. T - Teaching
3. O - Organization
4. P - Peer

It means in both cases that the requirements of the affected people must be satisfied basically within the framework of her acute stress reaction. What is necessary further are: safety, silences, the satisfaction of basic needs – first control over biological stress reactions search for natural resources, safe return in the own social networks and environment.

## 3 The PFA Core Actions

There are eight core actions of PFA according to Brymer et al. (2006):

1. Contact and Engagement. The goal is to respond to contact initiated by survivors or initiate contacts in a non-intrusive, compassionate manner.

2. Safety and Comfort. The goal is to enhance immediate and ongoing safety, and provide physical and emotional comfort.
3. Stabilisation (if needed). The goal is to calm and orient emotionally overwhelmed or disoriented survivors. All of the stress/anxiety reactions are NORMAL human reactions to a terrible incident. The use of "calming response" technique helps to fulfil the human needs.
4. Information gathering current needs and concerns. The goal is to identify immediate needs/concerns, gather additional information; give tailored PFA interventions.
5. Practical assistance. The goal is to offer practical help to survivors in addressing immediate needs and concerns.
6. Connection with social supports. The goal is to help establish brief and/or ongoing contacts with primary support persons and other sources of support, including family members, friends, and community helping resources.
7. Information on coping. The goal is to provide information about stress reactions and coping to reduce distress and promote adaptive functioning.
8. Linkage with collaborative services. The goal is to link survivors with available services needed at the time or in the future.

These actions and strategies should be part of learning psychological first aid. Where can this be learned? What is to determine in times without disaster? We cannot come to international disaster tourism to have practical training. So what can be done to teach and learn PFA?

## 4 How We Can Learn PFA

One can give a concise answer to this question. The best opportunity to learn PFA is in a crisis intervention team in times without disaster. There are also further education courses in Disaster Psychology and bachelor and master classes with project weeks and practical. Here we assume scientifically founded curricular further education and study programs. But also books and special literature are helpful. It can be recommended in the German-speaking part of the world, such as Kröger (2013), Perren-Klingler (1995, 2001, 2015), Gerngross and Guttmann (2014), and Lasogga and Gasch (2011). Other international authors have particular interest too, such as Everly and Mitchell (2001); Mitchell, Everly, Müller-Lange (2005); and Mitchell, George, Everly, Igl, Müller-Lange (1998).

The other way to learn what is essential to give PFA is given in training of the person centred approach by Carl Rogers (1983) and the Rosenberg's approach (2005) to nonviolent communication. In both approaches, communication training takes place, which seems to educate important basics of PFA. Notably, the underlying attitudes towards the person and basis communication skills are essential in the context of Disaster Psychology too.

Other online resources can be mentioned at the end: the PFA-online training approach of the National Child Traumatic Stress Network (NCTSN). PFA online education resources include a mostly interactive course that puts the participant in the role of a provider in a post-disaster scene. One can learn the core goals of PFA. Such a course features innovative activities, video demonstrations, and mentor tips from trauma experts and survivors. PFA online also offers a Learning Community where participants can share about experiences using PFA in the field, receive guidance during times of disaster, and obtain additional resources (see also NCTSN Learning Center).

Further online resource and information can be obtained from the National Center for PTSD of the US, the National Child Traumatic Stress Network (NCTSN) and the Psychological First Aid: Field Operations Guide 2nd Edition, and the International Critical Incident Stress Foundation.

## 5 Conclusions

There are many more programs, step by step strategies and core concepts for learning of PFA which can be used in self-learning and online training environment successfully for introduction in PFA. The "learning by doing" procedure in the local crisis intervention teams seems the best opportunity to learn PFA. Disaster Psychology training should belong to the basic skills trainings of psychologists and should be included in psychology training programs all over the world.

## 6 Affiliations

Prof. Dr. Konrad Reschke
Institution/address: University of Leipzig, Institute of Psychology, Neumarkt 9-19, 04109 Leipzig.
E-mail: konrad.reschke@web.de

M. Sc. Anar Bikadamova
Institution: Al Farabi Kazakh National University, Almaty, Kazakhstan.
Address: 71 al-Farabi Ave., Almaty, Republic of Kazakhstan, 050040.
E-mail: anarmilitary@mail.ru

M. Sc. Gulzat Sarbassova
Institution: Al Farabi Kazakh National University, Almaty, Kazakhstan
Address: 71 al-Farabi Ave., Almaty, Republic of Kazakhstan, 050040
E-mail: 85gulzat@mail.ru

## 7 References

Brymer, M., Jacobs, A., Layne, C., Pynoos, R., Ruzek, J., Steinberg, A., ... Watson, P. (2006). *Psychological first aid: Field operations guide 2nd edition.* Retrieved on September 14, 2010 from https://www.nctsn.org/sites/default/files/resources//pfa_field_operations_guide.pdf

Everly, G. S., & Mitchell, J. T. (2001). *CISM – Stressmanagement nach kritischen Ereignissen – ein neuer Versorgungsstandard bei Notfällen, Krisen und Katastrophen.* Wien: Facultas Wuv Universitätsverlag.

Gerngross, J., & Guttmann, G. (2014). *Notfallpsychologie und psychologisches Krisenmanagement.* Stuttgart: Schattauer.

Kröger, C. (2013). *Psychologische erste Hilfe.* Göttingen: Hogrefe.

Lasogga, G., & Gasch, B., (2011). *Notfallpsychologie.* Berlin: Springer.

Mitchell, J. T., Everly, G. S., & Müller-Lange, J. (2005). *Critical Incident Stress Management. Handbuch Einsatznachsorge.* Ederwecht: Stumpf & Kossendey Verlag.

Mitchell, J. T., George S., Everly, G. S., Igl, A., & Müller-Lange, J. (1998). *Streßbearbeitung nach belastenden Ereignissen. Zur Prävention psychischer Traumatisierung.* Edewecht: Stumpf & Kossendey Verlag.

Norris, F. H., Friedman, M. J., & Watson, P. J. (2002). 60,000 disaster victims speak: Part II. Summary and implications of the disaster mental health research. *Psychiatry, 65*(3), 240–260.

Perren-Klingler, G. (1995). *Trauma – Vom Schrecken des Einzelnen zu den Ressourcen der Gruppe.* Bern: Paul Haupt.

Perren-Klingler, G. (2001). *Debriefing – Erste Hilfe durch das Wort.* Bern: Paul Haupt.

Perren-Klingler, G. (2015). *Psychische Gesundheit und Katastrophe.* Berlin: Springer.

Rogers, C. (1983). *Die klientenzentrierte Gesprächspsychotherapie. Client-Centered Therapy.* Frankfurt am Main: Fischer Verlag GmbH.

Rosenberg, M. B. (2005). *Kinder einfühlend ins Leben begleiten: Elternschaft im Licht der gewaltfreien Kommunikation.* Paderborn: Junfermannsche Verlagsbuchhandlung.

Hamidreza Khankeh & Elham Sepahvand
# Concept Analysis of Bystander Effect in Road Traffic Injuries: A Hybrid Model

**Abstract:** The bystander effect that occurs at the scene of traffic accidents and emergencies can affect individuals' helping behavior. In this respect, several definitions have been provided to clarify and develop this concept. In the present study, the bystander effect occurring at the scene of traffic accidents in the Iranian context was analyzed. In this study, the concept analysis of the bystander effect was performed using a hybrid method recommended by Schwartz-Barcott in three phases (theoretical, fieldwork, and final analysis). Within the theoretical phase, a literature review was conducted employing different databases, and the related studies were analyzed. In the fieldwork phase, interviews were carried out with eight medical emergency personnel followed by qualitative content analysis of the transcriptions. Finally, in the last phase, an overall analysis was performed to come up with a clear definition of the given concept. In the final analysis phase, the following definition was achieved by integrating the two theoretical and fieldwork phases: "The bystander effect is a phenomenon occurring at the scene of traffic accidents and, in particular, emergencies. Within this phenomenon, the presence of bystanders at the scene can reduce the likelihood of individuals offering help to the injured. Observing the unstable condition of the injured and the fear of secondary damage also causes the bystander to stay out of the scene. Moreover, each bystander assumes others responsible for helping the injured. Influence from others' interpretations of the situation similarly helps with reinforcing this behavior." The study results could pave the way for further studies to develop the given concept in different cultures and also help to design a tool for further assessment of this phenomenon.

**Keywords:** bystander effect, medical emergencies, traffic accidents, hybrid model

## 1 Introduction

The bystander effect is a socio-psychological phenomenon in which the bystander does not offer help to the victims when other people are present at the scene (Latané & Darley, 1970). The bystander effect is also defined as a situation wherein they hesitate to assume any responsibility for helping the injured at the scene of an emergency and do not tend to participate because they feel other people at the scene would undertake such responsibilities (Schneider, Gruman, & Coutts, 2011). Numerous situational factors, such as the presence of others, similar involvement in the past, the appearance of the injured, and a sense of guilt could predict the pattern of the bystander's intervention and help behavior (Mason & Allen, 1976). In Mason and Allen's study, the bystander effect was defined as a case of inhibiting helping behavior due to the presence of people at the scene and the nonemergency state of the situation (Mason & Allen, 1976). Gottlieb & Carver (1980) also defined the bystander effect as follows: "When the bystanders at the scene are not acquainted with each other, they have no face-to-face interactions with and tend to withdraw from the scene; therefore, the speed of response to the emergency situation is reduced".

The bystander effect phenomenon has been examined in several studies, and the given concept has been defined in various ways, which might be due to differences in the background and culture of a wide range of communities studied. In their investigations regarded the presence of people at the scene of accidents, the one of the obstacles of pre-hospital care provided to the injured (Alinia, Khankeh, Maddah, & Negarandeh, 2015; Haghparast-Bidgoli, Hasselberg, Khankeh, Khorasani-Zavareh, & Johansson, 2010; Khankeh, Khorasani-Zavareh, & Masoumi, 2012; Khorasani-Zavareh, Khankeh, Mohammadi, Laflamme, Bikmoradi, & Haglund, 2009). According to those studies, as the number of bystanders on the scene increased, the likelihood of people's interventions was raised, and care was hindered accordingly.

Given the importance of the concept of the bystander effect and that of the background and structure governing the scene of traffic accidents, which have resulted in different meanings in such a structure, it seems necessary to develop the concept in order to understand it better. As one of the approaches to concept analysis in clinical practice, the hybrid approach is appropriate for investigating the concept of the bystander effect in the Iranian context in light of participants' experiences.

## 2 Materials and Methods

A hybrid model was used to analyze the bystander effect as recommended by Schwartz-Barcott (as cited in Madden, 1990). The model provides a method for conceptualising and clarifying the concept as well as developing theories. In the hybrid model, deductive and inductive methods are combined. This model, often used in nursing, consists of three phases: theoretical analysis, fieldwork, and final analysis. In the hybrid model, theoretical and practical studies are combined.

## 3 Results

### 3.1 Results of the theoretical phase

At the end of the theoretical phase, the characteristics of the concept were identified. These characteristics are indispensable parts of the concept without which a clear picture of the concept could not be presented (Latané & Rodin, 1969). After an extensive review of the studies (see Table 1), the following characteristics of the bystander effect were identified: *Presence of strangers, pluralistic ignorance, diffusion of responsibility, social influence, and self-safety.*

Table 1. Some Studies into the Bystander Effect Phenomenon at the Scene of an Emergency

| Author | Background under study | Characteristics | Antecedents | Consequences |
| --- | --- | --- | --- | --- |
| Hortensius, Schutter, & Gelder (2016) | Effect of group size on helping behavior in an emergency | Social influence of the presence of others, observing the person, and increasing helping behavior | Being observed by others, strong emotional reactions to the situation | **Increasing helping behavior** |
| van Bommel, van Prooijen, Elffers, & Van Lange (2012) | Bystander effect and increasing general self-awareness | Increasing general self-awareness and increasing helping behavior | Concerns about others' perceptions of behavior, sense of responsibility, the presence of the camera, or fear of being labelled | **Increasing helping behavior and increasing the cost-effectiveness of a behavior** |
| Tice & Baumeister (1985) | Relationship between personality and gender and their effects on helping behavior in emergency situations | Individual differences and personality traits reduce the instances of helping behavior | Presence of people, lack of self-confidence, lack of sense of independence, being male, personality traits | **Apathy and reluctance to help** |
| Darley & Latané (1968) | Bystander intervention in emergency situations | Presence of others in an emergency reduces the level of individual responsibility | Fear of feeling embarrassed in front of others, the presence of males | **Reluctance to help** |
| Latané & Rodin (1969) | Effect of the presence of friends and strangers on the intervention of bystanders at the scene | Diffusion of responsibility, pluralistic ignorance, and presence of strangers | Individual experiences, not taking the situation seriously, predilection | **Worsening of the situation of the injured** |

(*continued on next page*)

Table 1. Continued

| Author | Background under study | Characteristics | Antecedents | Consequences |
|---|---|---|---|---|
| Mason & Allen (1976) | Bystander effect as a function of emergency | Avoiding help due to the presence of people and when the situation is a nonemergency | Vague situation and nonemergency conditions | **Staying out of the scene without offering help** |
| Bickman (1971) | Bystander's ability to intervene in emergency situations | Inability to provide help and shifting responsibility onto someone else | Lack of knowledge, personal judgment, and interpreting the situation as a nonemergency | **Avoiding intervening in the scene and providing help to the injured** |
| Bickman (1972) | Social influence of the diffusion of responsibility in an emergency | Gaining influence from others and regarding the situation as nonemergency | Individual's interpretations of emergency and others' behavior present at the scene | **Avoiding helping others** |
| Gottlieb & Carver (1980) | Bystander effect and face-to-face interactions | Lack of face-to-face interactions reduces the speed of response to emergency situations | Individual's behavior performed in an emergency | **Increased costs** |
| Zoccola & Dickerson (2012) | Embarrass-ment and performing no helping behavior | Fear of embarrassment in front of others and reducing helping behavior | Bitter experiences of the past, social pressures | **Staying away from the scene and being an observer** |

## 3.2 Final definition of the theoretical phase

The bystander effect is a social psychological phenomenon in which an individual fail to provide help to the victims at the scene when other people are present. According to this effect, as the number of bystanders at the scene increases, the likelihood of offering help to the injured is reduced. When a person is alone at the scene of the accident, they feel fully responsible for providing help to the injured, recognize the scene as an emergency based on their experience and interpretation, and consequently intervene. In contrast, with the presence of other bystanders on the scene, this sense of responsibility is diminished, and the person influenced by others' reactions and interpretations might interpret the situation as a nonemergency and thus feel reluctant to offer help.

## 3.3 Results of the fieldwork phase

One of the characteristics obtained in the fieldwork phase was that the people were strangers. When the bystander and the injured are relatives, the former are more likely to show emotional reactions, and their interventions are more tangible. They may even come into conflict with others and the medical emergency personnel for not offering help. These are some main characteristics which explored from field work: *Unstable condition of the injured, lack of awareness, gaining influence from certain individuals and pluralistic ignorance, and presence of medical emergency personnel.*

## 3.4 Final definition resulting from the integration of the theoretical and fieldwork phases

The bystander effect is a phenomenon occurring at the scene of traffic accidents and emergencies in general. In this phenomenon, the bystander, present at the scene of the accident, observes the situation. First, the bystander feels obliged to offer help to the injured, but the unstable condition of the injured, as well as the fear of secondary damage, cause them to withdraw from the scene. In addition, the presence of other bystanders at the scene makes the initial bystander deny any responsibility for helping the injured and shift it onto others. The behavior is reinforced by the influence of others' interpretations of a situation as being an emergency or a nonemergency.

# 4 Discussion and Conclusion

This study aimed to clarify the concept of the bystander effect occurring at the scene of traffic accidents and presented various characteristics of this phenomenon. The results of the literature review and fieldwork phases showed that the bystander effect repeatedly occurs at emergency scenes. In this phenomenon, as the number of bystanders on the scene increases, the instances of helping behavior decrease, and each regards others as responsible for providing help and intervention. In such a situation, one or more persons might intervene as the leader or manager of the scene, and their perceptions of the scene and of the need to offer help to the injured could influence others' perceptions. The bystander effect is more likely to occur when the people at the scene are strangers with little knowledge of first aid (Bickman, 1971; Darley, 1968; Latané & Nida, 1981).

According to these results, the bystander effect is a phenomenon in which a person is placed in the position of offering help to the injured. The presence of others at the scene, the unstable condition of the injured, lack of knowledge, and being influenced by other's behaviors are among factors that affect denying responsibility and shifting it onto medical emergency personnel, thus refraining from offering help to the injured. The analysis of the bystander effect indicated that the concept includes a set of behaviors and characteristics partly guided by cultural background and context. Further development of this concept could help expand the existing body of knowledge in the field of pre-hospital emergency and develop models and theories about traffic accidents. Developing a context-bound tool based on the results of this study is recommended.

# 5 Affiliations

Prof. Dr. Hamidreza Khankeh
Institution/address: University of Social Welfare and Rehabilitation Sciences Tehran, Evin, Student Blvd, Kodakyar Alley, Postal code: 1985713834.
E-mail: hamid.khankeh@ki.se

Dr. Elham Sepahvand
Institution/address: University of Social Welfare and Rehabilitation Sciences Tehran, Evin, Student Blvd, Kodakyar Alley, Postal code: 1985713834.
E-mail: el.sepahvand@yahoo.com

# 6 References

Alinia, S., Khankeh, H. R, Maddah, S. S. B., & Negarandeh, R. (2015). Barriers of pre-hospital services in road traffic injuries in Tehran: The viewpoint of service providers. *International Journal of Community Based Nursing and Midwifery*, *3*(4), 272.

Bickman, L. (1971). The effect of another bystander's ability to help on bystander intervention in an emergency. *Journal of Experimental Social Psychology*, *7*(3), 367–379.

Bickman, L. (1972). Social influence and diffusion of responsibility in an emergency. *Journal of Experimental Social Psychology*, *8*(5), 438–445.

Darley, J. M., & Latane, B. (1968). Bystander intervention in emergencies: diffusion of responsibility. *Journal of Personality and Social Psychology*, *8*(4), 377.

Gottlieb, J., & Carver, C. S. (1980). Anticipation of future interaction and the bystander effect. *Journal of Experimental Social Psychology*, *16*(3), 253–260.

Haghparast-Bidgoli, H., Hasselberg, M., Khankeh, H. R., Khorasani-Zavareh, D., & Johansson, E. (2010). Barriers and facilitators to provide effective pre-hospital trauma care for road traffic injury victims in Iran: A grounded theory approach. *BMC Emergency Medicine*, *10*(1), 1.

Hortensius, R., Schutter, D. J., & Gelder, B. (2016). Personal distress and the influence of bystanders on responding to an emergency. *Cognitive, Affective, & Behavioral Neuroscience*, *16*(4), 672–688.

Khankeh, H. R., Khorasani-Zavareh, D., & Masoumi, G. (2012). Why the Prominent Improvement in Prehospital Medical Response in Iran Couldn't Decrease the Number of Death Related Road Traffic Injuries. *Trauma & Treatment, 1*(4).

Khorasani-Zavareh, D., Khankeh, H. R., Mohammadi, R., Laflamme, L., Bikmoradi, A., & Haglund, B. J. (2009). Post-crash management of road traffic injury victims in Iran. Stakeholders' views on current barriers and potential facilitators. *BMC Emergency Medicine, 9*(1), 8.

Latané, B., & Darley, J. M. (1970). *The unresponsive bystander: Why doesn't he help?* New York: Prentice Hall.

Latané, B., & Nida, S. (1981). Ten years of research on group size and helping. *Psychological Bulletin, 89*(2), 308.

Latané, B., & Rodin, J. (1969). A lady in distress: Inhibiting effects of friends and strangers on bystander intervention. *Journal of Experimental Social Psychology, 5*(2), 189–202.

Madden, B. P. (1990). The hybrid model for concept development: Its value for the study of therapeutic alliance. *Advances in Nursing Science, 12*(3), 75–87.

Mason, D., & Allen, B. P. (1976). The bystander effect as a function of ambiguity and emergency character. *The Journal of Social Psychology, 100*(1), 145–146.

Schneider, F. W., Gruman, J. A., & Coutts, L. M. (2011). *Applied Social Psychology: Understanding and addressing social and practical problems.* Los Angeles: Sage.

Tice, D. M., & Baumeister, R. F. (1985). Masculinity inhibits helping in emergencies: Personality does predict the bystander effect. *Journal of Personality and Social Psychology, 49*(2), 420.

van Bommel, M., van Prooijen, J.-W., Elffers, H., & Van Lange, P. A. (2012). Be aware to care: Public self-awareness leads to a reversal of the bystander effect. *Journal of Experimental Social Psychology, 48*(4), 926–930.

Zoccola, P. M., & Dickerson, S. S. (2012). Assessing the relationship between rumination and cortisol: A review. *Journal of Psychosomatic Research, 73*(1), 1–9.

Juliet Roudini, Hamidreza Khankeh, Evelin Witruk, Abbas Ebadi,
Konrad Reschke, & Marcus Stueck

# Dimensions of Community Mental Health Preparedness of Disasters in Iran

**Abstract:** Over the past twenty-six years, some disasters, affected people and economic damages as a consequence are increasing worldwide Asian countries have always been among the top ten affected ones by various kinds of disasters. Iran is one of the countries which is prone to many natural disasters such as earthquakes, floods, drought and storms. It seems necessary to study the mental health of the community in disaster situations to endorse their health and prevent disorders as well as care planning. Therefore, a clear understanding of the community mental health preparedness is necessary based on experiences and perceptions of involved people. The purpose of this article was a subjective and comprehensive description of community mental health preparedness in disasters. A qualitative inductive content analysis method was exploited. Participants included 14 experts and lay people. Data were collected through in-depth, semi-structured interviews. All interviews were transcribed and data analysis was accomplished based on qualitative inductive content analysis principles. Data were explored using content analysis and found five categories, including 1) cultural values and beliefs, 2) risk beliefs, 3) mental preparedness in disasters, 4) psychological process, and 5) trust. Mental health preparedness is a multifactorial phenomenon that requires a clear understanding and definition of perceived threats (risk), public trust in social structure and formal and informal supportive organization. This preparedness involves proportional, mental, social, familial, religious beliefs, and cultural sensitive along with the ability to handle the mentally disastrous situation which can be measured after concept analysis and tool development process.

**Keywords:** content analysis, community, mental health, preparedness, disasters

## 1 Introduction

Natural disasters have affected the whole world throughout history with numerous effects on the community. For many people, catastrophes constitute a personal tragedy that involves the loss of health, properties, loved ones and their occupations and resources. According to the definition of the International Federation of Red Cross and Red Crescent Societies (IFRC), a disaster is an unexpected, catastrophic event that seriously interrupts the functioning of a community or society and causes human and economic or environmental losses that exceed the community's or society's capacity to use its resources. Iran has a high level of exposure to numerous disaster risks. Because it is located in one of the aridest areas of the world, droughts, earthquakes, floods, sand and dust storms, and forest fires increasingly affect different parts of Iran.

Posttraumatic stress disorder (PTSD) is the most commonly identified disorder that happens after experiencing a dangerous event (The National Institute of Mental Health, 2017). PTSD is considered as re-experiencing of the traumatic event, avoidance, numbing and hyperarousal. Depression is the second most commonly observed psychological disorder in survivors of disasters followed by various problems with anxiety (Graham, 2012; Norris, Perilla, Riad, Kaniasty, & Lavizzo, 1999).

Studies showed that providing only medical and financial support in disasters cannot decrease the long-term psychological and mental effects of disasters (Krug et al., 1998; Norris, Friedman, & Watson, 2002). In the human-made and natural disasters with a focus on mental health difficulties, there is a lack of a well-defined concept of mental health preparedness for disasters. In Asia mental illness such as a PTSD, major depressive disorder and anxiety are due to a lack of mental health preparedness and insufficient knowledge and practices; concerning the mental health preparedness (Udomratn, 2008). In previous research, the absence of mental health preparedness information on vulnerable peoples such as children, women, people living with disabilities and the elderly have been indicated (Black, 1982; Schonfeld & Gurwitch, 2009; Sharma, Kumar, & Raja, 2015).

## 2 The importance of Preparedness and Exploring this Concept in Iranian Context

Iran is one of the most disaster-prone countries in the world (Khankeh, Khorasani-Zacareh, Johanson, Mohammadi, Ahmadi, & Mohammadi, 2011) and for many of reasons, Iran and other Asian countries do not have appropriate preparations for dealing and coping with disasters and their consequences. According to the World Health Organization (WHO), the situation of Bam earthquake in south-eastern Iran on December 26 in 2003, all of the survivors required extensive psychological counselling, and psychiatric treatment and around 40% of the affected population developed PTSD (WHO, 2014). At that time, due to a lack of proper training, awareness, and preparedness, some people were psychologically affected by the incident and were emotionally uncontrollable.

The importance of mental health preparedness in disasters is increasingly being documented as a superiority for community mental health emergency in different researches (Davidson & McFarlane, 2006; Meredith et al., 2011; Pfefferbaum & North, 2013). Mental health is closely linked with physical health, behavior health, recruitment, educational proficiency, crime reduction (Herrman & Jané-Llopis, 2012; Friedli & WHO, 2009). Mental health preparedness supports people and communities to reach their potential and also increase their ability (Patel, Fisher, Hetrick, & McGorry, 2007). Therefore, the communities must be prepared psychologically to cope with disasters to avoid the long-term psychological effects. Hence, with the present lack of knowledge about mental health and mental preparedness in the incidents at the community level, the current study aims to explore this important phenomenon through the perception and experiences of people.

# 3 Methodological framework

## 3.1 Study Design

Community mental health Preparedness is subjective, culturally sensitive and context bond, therefore, a qualitative approach was an appropriate method to understand and explore this phenomenon (Ranjbar, Khankeh, Khorasani Zavareh, Zargham-Boroujeni, & Johansson, 2015). The content analysis method was selected for reaching a deep understanding of community perspectives and their limitations about mental health preparedness in disaster situations. The analysis distracted the experiences of expert and non-expert group in several categories. Data were collected by concentrating on interviewees' perspectives. By using an inductive approach, codes were set to decrease volumes of verbal into more manageable data to identify patterns and gain insight.

## 3.2 Study Participants

Considering the content analysis and the phenomena of mental health preparedness, the samples were selected from among experts in disasters and emergencies and the survivors ($n$ = 14).

## 3.3 Data Gathering

Semi-structured interviews were conducted at the data gathering tool. The interview guide included general and specific questions were administered to direct the interview.

## 3.4 Data Analysis

A qualitative content analysis was used for the interpretation of interviews. This method was used to recognise both the manifest and latent content of the text (Graneheim & Lundman, 2004).

After the data analysis was transcribed and checked by the experts, the reduced meaning units were condensed into codes, and subcategories and categories were emerged based on likenesses and differences in content. Similarities and differences of insights of participants were recognised. Finally, a combination of categories was done by connecting them to the themes and by using methods including immersion in the data, reviewing memos, making descriptive sentences and drawing diagrams.

## 3.5 Trustworthiness and Ethical Considerations

Specific strategies were used to ensure the trustworthiness of data. They include a) peer review; meaning that in several times data interpretation was checked by other researchers in this field), and b) member check by participants to recheck the data and our understandings from data which were revised and confirmed by them.

# 4 Results

Based on the content analysis, the attributes of the data of mental health preparedness for disasters can be divided into five major categories and 12 subcategories and 31 codes which the major categories including 1) cultural values and beliefs, 2) risk beliefs, 3) mental health preparedness in disasters, 4) psychological process, and 5) trust. These categories and subcategories are described in the next sections.

## 4.1 Cultural Values and Beliefs

### 4.1.1 Spiritual Beliefs and Disaster Beliefs

Religions and beliefs play significant roles because of their supporting defines for disasters.

### 4.1.2 Thankfulness, Determinism, Reliance, Fatalism, Punishment, Destiny, Projection

In this study, "cultural values and beliefs" was one of the challenges which were extracted from experiences and perceptions of the participants and divided into two subcategories: Spiritual Beliefs and Disaster Beliefs. Religions and beliefs play a significant role because of their supporting defines for disasters. It can help people deal with why something overwhelming occurred to them: they can turn to their beliefs for relief and support. However, to the disaster experts and management, beliefs can seem unusable – even to the point of uselessly increasing people's exposure to hazard.

On the other hand, most of the experts mentioned that this belief should be more considered because people are not prepared for confronting a disaster due to spiritual beliefs.

## 4.2 Risk Belief

This concept contains two subcategories: feeling and understanding the risk and lack of risk believe. Another theme frequently discussed by the experts was feeling and understanding the risk, they are:

### 4.2.1 Lack of Risk Understanding

The current study shows that communities do not have same risk understanding of disaster and disaster risk management rather than concentrating on what limits communities' ability to decrease their risk, instead should emphasises on understanding risk between different group of communities.

### 4.2.2 Lack of risk perception

There was a low level of awareness among the lay people; concerning the threat that disasters represent to them and their community.

### 4.2.3 Temporary Attention and Impact of Severity and Magnitude on Attention

It is upsetting to wonder how the culture and media seem to take short-term attention in disasters. Factually, the media has always had a temporary attention span for disasters

### 4.2.4 Lack of risk believing in young people

The number of children and young people affected by catastrophes and emergencies is anticipated to increase threefold over the next years due to climate change, disasters, and population growth. Therefore, it is important that communities, especially young people, become better prepared for disasters and disaster mental health preparedness is significant for reducing the vulnerability of young people in disasters.

### 4.2.5 Lack of Acceptance of Disasters and Ignorance

People refuse to live in fear of the unknown; therefore, they do not want to accept a disaster risk in future.

### 4.2.6 Lack of Knowledge and Belief of different kinds of Disaster Risk

Most people do not have sufficient knowledge about disasters, its effects, and think that just because a disaster happens.

### 4.2.7 Lack of Experience in Emergency Workers

Most participants mentioned that emergency management at different levels came to their duties with practically no experience in handling a catastrophe.

### 4.2.8 Lack of Anticipation

It is significant to ask what plan we can have to anticipate disasters, to decrease their influence, and to enable the affected communities to recover through proper preparedness and resilience.

## 4.3 Mental Health Preparedness in Disasters

### 4.3.1 Planning and Strategies

In a disaster event, many staff and volunteers come immediately to deliver mental health and psychosocial support to the affected people, but they typically come with their specific agenda. They come from different socio-economic and cultural levels, background and even language than the affected people. Therefore, they carry, unlike values and views.

### 4.3.2 Education

A social relief worker in a disastrous situation is not well prepared to help people in that condition. It is necessary to educate this group of the people to how to handle their feeling at a catastrophic situation and at the same time be helpful for affected people.

### 4.3.3 Social Participation

Disaster mental health preparedness is not a completely individual effort as social participation and networks can also develop it. Efforts to help disaster mental health preparedness and risk reduction often accentuate the importance of people participating.

### 4.3.4 Presence or Absence of Mental Health Preparedness

#### 4.3.4.1 The existence of Individual Safety and Preparedness, Lack of Mental Health Preparedness

Catastrophic events like earthquakes can strike rapidly and without warning; making families to evacuate their neighbourhoods or limiting them to their households. Understanding what to do is individual's best defence and responsibility. It is unfeasible to think that one can be wholly prepared psychologically, for such a traumatic incident. Awareness, Sensitization, Knowledge and Finding Information

#### 4.3.4.2 Curiosity and Sensitivity, Awareness, Knowledge and Finding Information

Psychological preparedness can be improved through the acquisition of specific psychological knowledge and strategies, and through being Sensitization to disastrous issues and acquiring information. We must consider that the community has a sense of curiosity about a disaster and it can be a good point to improve this sense appropriately.

## 4.4 Psychological Process

The psychological process is related to the psychological effects and reactions, coping strategies, and its disorders. The impact of exposure to a disaster is varies, especially to individual characteristics. In general, those that confronted to a disaster show increased the level of posttraumatic stress disorder (PTSD), major depression, acute stress disorder, panic disorder, substance use disorder and anxiety disorder.

Faith and religion and their interventions were already rooted in the communities so that people could turn to their faith during the disaster. Therefore, people after disasters were more resilient, and they could get back to their normal life rapidly because of these cultural coping strategies.

The role of the clergymen in providing psychosocial and mental health support was also viewed as significant by some participants.

## 4.5 Trust

Issues related to this theme are about trust to the structures, such as lack of trust to the organizations, the relief workers, the media, and the psychologists. Trust is the basis of all human connections. In disaster risk management, a powerful communication strategy is probably an effective way to expand trust relationships. We can develop trust building by clear, open and efficient communication.

Using media will be increased during a disaster among people who are either directly or indirectly affected. According to study results, there is a lack of trust in the data exchanged via media and social media and this lack of trust may expressively prevent decision-making by emergency management and community during disasters.

# 5 Discussion

This study has shown that the related concepts are 1) cultural values and beliefs, 2) risk beliefs, 3) mental preparedness in disasters, 4) psychological process and 5) trust.

Based on this study, cultural values and beliefs mean the collection of perception and reaction of the community to a disaster like a thankfulness, determinism, reliance and fatalism. In our study, we revealed that beliefs are related to disaster risk because it can provide a stage for the support community to cope with the impacts of incidents and educating peoples about risk reduction.

Regarding risk beliefs, people have the right to know the risks that they are confronting in the future, and according to their knowledge be aware that how to be able to take actions. It means that recognising and understanding disaster risk is the underpinning for disaster preparedness and it is significant to identify which aspects affect the degree of acceptance of people to the risks.

Due to a lack of community mental health preparedness, we need to educate people on a different level and also increase their social participation. We need to improve Individual Safety and Preparedness. Psychological preparedness can be improved through the acquisition of specific psychological knowledge and strategies, and through being Sensitization to disastrous issues and acquiring information.

Regarding the psychological process and reactions to disasters, according to our literature review, most people can experience mild distress reactions. In our fieldwork stage, participants indicated that traditional coping strategies like faith and religion beliefs, family involvement for accepting incident were necessary to help them to cope with the impact of disasters.

The findings of our study showed that there was a lack of trust between communities and emergency centres and related organizations. A significant category that merged by many participants was mistrust to media, government, utilities and other organizations and these organizations have less information regarding other's activities and responsibilities of expertise and actions for operation. This lack of understanding can lead to mistrust among administrations and improbable expectations of operations, which can, in turn, lead to an undervaluing of the immediate tasks and the expertise required doing them.

# 6 Conclusion

According to our qualitative finding we reached to this definition of mental health preparedness "mental preparedness in natural disasters is a complex and relative concept which is dependent on public trust to structures and organizations, official and unofficial supportive sources. It is based on this trust that people organize their supportive actions for themselves and their families. This trust can lead to positive, psychological reactions".

Proposing this definition of Community mental health preparedness in disasters which is based on the theoretical and field work stage definition of the concept has two main applications in developing the instrumentation.

The mental preparedness planning of disaster management must include the development of existing mental health facilities. The healthcare employees in primary healthcare can be used to deliver psychological first aid which is traditionally and culturally suitable and acceptable. The satisfactory method of disaster preparedness in mental health is to have a strong community mental health system.

Therefore, the community must learn about how a catastrophe situation is likely to be experienced, how they can support in handling one's stress and anxiety and general psychological reactions, and how an effective decision can be made at imminent disaster threat. The results of this study can be used to assess community mental health preparedness and develop some interventions like training programs to increase community mental preparedness in any different group of society. The results of the qualitative section can be useful in health sector planning and policy.

# 7 Affiliations

Dr. Juliet Roudini
Institution/address: Institute of Psychology, University of Leipzig, Neumarkt 9-19, 04109 Leipzig, Germany.
E-mail: juliet.roudini@studserv.uni-leipzig.de

Prof. Dr. Hamidreza Khankeh
Institution/address 1: Department of Health in Emergency and Disaster, and Nursing, the University of Social Welfare and Rehabilitation Science, Tehran, Iran.
Institution/address 2: Department of Clinical Science and Education, Karolinska Institute, Södersjukhuset (KI SÖS) Stockholm, Sweden.
E-mail: hamid.khankeh@ki.se

Prof. Dr. Evelin Witruk
Institution/address: Institute of Psychology, University of Leipzig, Neumarkt 9-19, 04109 Leipzig, Germany.
E-mail: witruk@uni-leipzig.de

Prof. Dr. Abbas Ebadi
Institution/address: Behavioral Sciences Research Center, Lifestyle Institute, Faculty of Nursing, Baqiyatallah University of Medical Sciences, Tehran, Iran.
E-mail: ebadi1347@yahoo.com

Prof. Dr. Konrad Reschke
Institution/address: Department of Clinical Psychology, Institute of Psychology, University of Leipzig, Neumarkt 9-19, 04109 Leipzig, Germany.
E-mail: reschke@uni-leipzig.de

Prof. Dr. Marcus Stueck
Institution/address: DPFA Academy for Work and Health, DPFA-Weiterbildung GmbH, Education Center Leipzig, Taeubschenweg 83, 04317 Leipzig, Germany.
Email: marcus.stueck@dpfa-hs.de

# 8 References

Black, D. (1982). Children and disaster. *British Medical Journal, 285*(6347), 989–990. doi: 10.1136/bmj.285.6347.989

Davidson, J. R., & McFarlane, A. C. (2006). The extent and impact of mental health problems after disaster. *Journal of Clinical Psychiatry, 67*(suppl 2), 9–14.

Friedli, L., & World Health Organization. (2009). *Mental health, resilience and inequalities.* Copenhagen: WHO Regional Office for Europe.

Graham, J. (2012, November 10). The emotional aftermath of Hurricane Sandy. New York: New York Times.

Graneheim, U., & Lundman, B. (2004). Qualitative content analysis in nursing research: Concepts, procedures and measures to achieve trustworthiness. *Nurse Education Today, 24*(2), 105–12. doi: 10.1016/j.nedt.2003.10.001

Herrman, H., & Jané-Llopis, E. (2012). The status of mental health promotion. *Public Health Reviews, 34*(2), 1–21. doi: 10.1007/ bf03391674

Khankeh, H. R., Khorasani-Zavareh, D., Johanson, E., Mohammadi, R., Ahmadi, F., & Mohammadi, R. (2011). Disaster health related challenges and requirements: A grounded theory study in Iran. *Prehospital and Disaster Medicine, 26*(3), 151–158. doi: 10.1017/s1049023x11006200

Krug, E. G., Kresnow, M., Peddicord, J. P., Dahlberg, L. L., Powell, K. E., Crosby, A. E., & Annest, J. L. (1998). Suicide after Natural Disasters. *New England Journal of Medicine, 338*(6), 373–378. doi: 10.1056/ nejm199802053380607

Meredith, L. S., Eisenman, D. P., Tanielian, T., Taylor, S. L., Basurto-Davila, R., Zazzali, J., ... Shields, S. (2011). Prioritizing "psychological" consequences for disaster preparedness and response: A framework for addressing the emotional, behavioral, and cognitive effects of patient surge in large scale disasters. *Disaster Medicine and Public Health Preparedness, 5*(01), 73–80. doi: 10.1001/dmp.2010.47

Norris, F. H., Friedman, M. J., & Watson, P. J. 60,000 Disaster victims speak; Part II: Summary and implications of the disaster mental health research. *Psychiatry: Interpersonal and Biological Processes, 65*(3), 240–260. doi: 10.1521/psyc.65.3.240.20169

Norris, F. H., Perilla, J. L., Riad, J. K., Kaniasty, K., & Lavizzo, F. A. (1999). Stability and change in stress, resources, and psychological distress following natural disaster: Findings from hurricane Andrew. *Anxiety, Stress & Coping, 12*(4), 363–396. doi: 10.1080/10615809908249317

Patel, V., Flisher, A. J., Hetrick, S., & McGorry, P. (2007). Mental health of young people: A global public-health challenge. *The Lancet, 369*(9569), 1302–13. doi: 10.1016/s0140-6736(07)60368-7

Pfefferbaum, B., & North, C. S. (2013). Assessing children's disaster reactions and mental health needs: screening and clinical evaluation. *The Canadian Journal of Psychiatry, 58*(3), 135–142. doi: 10.1177/070674371305800303318

Ranjbar, M., Khankeh, H., Khorasani Zavareh, D., ZarghamBoroujeni, A., & Johansson E. (2015). Challenges in conducting qualitative research in health: A conceptual paper. *Iranian Journal of Nursing and Midwifery Research, 20*(6), 635. doi: 10.4103/1735-9066.170010

Schonfeld, D. J., & Gurwitch, R. H. (2009). Addressing disaster mental health needs of children: Practical guidance for pediatric emergency health care providers. *Clinical Pediatric Emergency Medicine, 10*(3), 208–215. doi: 10.1016/j.cpem.2009.06.002

Sharma, R., Kumar, V., & Raja, D. (2015). Disaster preparedness amongst women, the invisible force of resilience: A study from Delhi, India. *International Journal of Health System and Disaster Management, 3*(3), 163. doi: 10.4103/2347-9019.157402

The National Institute of Mental Health. (2017). *Post-Traumatic Stress Disorders (PTSD)*. Retrieved on May 23, 2018 from https://www.nimh.nih.gov/health/publications/post-traumatic-stress-disorder-ptsd/ptsd-508-05172017_38054.pdf

Udomratn, P. (2008). Mental health and the psychosocial consequences of natural disasters in Asia. *International Review of Psychiatry, 20*(5), 441–444. doi: 10.1080/09540260802397487

World Health Organization. (2014). *Health services must stop leaving older people behind.* Geneva: World Health Organization.

Johanna Sophie von Lieres

# Mental Well-Being and Protective Factors in Vulnerable Groups: Victims of the 2004 Tsunami in Kerala, South India, and Disadvantaged Rural Populations in North India

**Abstract:** Vulnerable population groups in India face many challenges, for example, social discrimination and economic disadvantages. They face the risk of poverty which prevents them from having their basic needs met. Accessing healthcare, education, proper nutrition, and having their human rights respected is not a given for these marginalised groups. In two research studies with two different vulnerable population groups in rural India, the author explored potential protective factors, which aid in maintaining mental well-being in spite of hardships. The first study was a quantitative cross-sectional comparative study with tsunami survivors in fishing villages in Kerala, India, who were still traumatised 2.5 years after the disaster. They were shown to be protected from psychological distress by Antonovsky's Sense of Coherence, perceived social support, and avoidance coping. The second study was a qualitative, explorative study with residents of disadvantaged rural communities in Northern India. Material wealth, education, and family, followed by religious/spiritual practices, to be the most salient sources of happiness or life satisfaction, which can be seen as protective factors. In both samples, social relations were crucial for mental well-being. Organizations or agencies concerned with village development should investigate, which protective factors are available and sought after in the respective village community and give priority to strengthening these.

**Keywords:** vulnerable groups, survivors of disasters, rural India, protective factors, mental well-being

## 1 Introduction

In this article, the author presents two examples of vulnerable populations: (1) the survivors of the 2004 Asian tsunami in fishing villages along the Western coastline of Kerala, South India, and (2) residents of economically deprived villages from six states in North India. For both populations, studies were conducted to explore protective factors which enhanced the participants' mental well-being and protected them from psychological distress.

Once the most important protective factors or factors enhancing mental well-being for a population are known, non-governmental organizations (NGOs) focusing on rural development know where to set priorities in their approach.

Any change in village people's living conditions needs to go hand in hand with an improved quality of life (QoL) or subjective well-being (SWB).

In many areas of lower to lower-middle income countries, poverty prevents meeting the most basic human needs. Those who fail to thrive economically and socially are the world's vulnerable populations. People from vulnerable groups are often marginalised and neglected since they lack effective advocacy. In rural India, examples of such vulnerable sections of society are the elderly, children and adolescents, and women. Another vulnerable group is victims of natural or man-made disasters such as cyclones, earthquakes, famines, war, terrorism and communal/ethnic strife (Goel, Agarwal, Ichhpujani, & Shrivastana, 2004).

Disaster victims have faced extreme disruption and great loss. Therefore, they are more prone to common mental illnesses due to increased mental distress (e.g., depression, anxiety, substance abuse, post-traumatic stress disorder [PTSD]). PTSD is not the main mental disorder resulting from a disaster but one of a range of common mental disorders, which become more prevalent after a disaster. Trauma and loss may (a) exacerbate previous mental illness (e.g., it may turn moderate depression into severe depression) and (b) cause a severe form of trauma-induced common mental disorder in some people (World Health Organization Regional Office for South-East Asia [WHO SEARO], 2005).

In India, 68.8% of the population live in rural areas (Census of India, 2011). India's villagers can be seen as a vulnerable group since they face poverty, illiteracy, malnutrition, and lack of basic facilities. The majority (75%) of rural households need to manage on less than Rupees 5,000 (65 Euro) a month. More than a quarter (26%) of rural households are below the poverty line (BPL). More than 50% of rural households do not own land and depend on casual labour. Data shows that 42% of rural women and 23% of rural men are illiterate (Socio-Economic Census, 2011). In 2006, 81% of children up to 3 years and 58% of women of reproductive age suffered from anaemia in rural areas (Mukunthan, 2015).

In light of these hardships that the people in rural India are facing, government schemes and NGOs are trying to alleviate the worst of the problems. One such NGO-based project is Amrita Self-Reliant Village (SeRVe), which is part of the deemed university Amrita Vishwa Vidyapeetham in Kerala, India. The Amrita Vishwa Vidyapeetham University is one of many institutions and humanitarian initiatives run by the Mata Amritanandamayi Math, an NGO led by the renowned humanitarian and spiritual leader Sri Mata Amritanandamayi Devi, also known as Amma (mother) to many. The Amrita SeRVe project has the goal to strengthen India's villages by simultaneously addressing seven focus areas: health, education, agriculture, income generation, water and sanitation, eco-friendly infrastructure, and self-empowerment.

## 2 Theoretical Background

All over the globe, there are people who benefit from the globalisation of markets and those who do not. A population's well-being can be defined by the Gross

Domestic Product (GDP) per capita and by life expectancy. The latter has increased significantly in lower to lower-middle income countries, even if GDP hasn't (Becker, Philipson, & Soares, 2003). In recent decades, however, the trend has gone from defining a nation's development by GDP and life expectancy or literacy rates alone to additionally assessing social and psychological factors of well-being. QoL research is investigating objective, as well as subjective components of an individual's well-being, whereas SWB research is focusing on a person's subjective experience of his or her life (Diener, 1984).

Objective determinants, such as material well-being, environmental factors, and having basic needs met (e.g., food, safe drinking water, shelter, education, healthcare), are important for QoL, as well as emotional and physical well-being (Schalock et al., 2002). Diener, Diener, and Diener (1995) investigated factors related to SWB across 55 nations and found that income in itself was not related to SWB beyond having one's basic needs met.

Not all members of vulnerable populations – who often lack the fulfilment of basic needs – despair, though, and not all survivors of disasters suffer from PTSD. Many people seem to survive a traumatic event unscathed. In the 1970s, the focus of mental health research shifted from pathology to competence or "resiliency" in the face of adverse situations. For example, Aaron Antonovsky (1979) wanted to identify the psychological, social, and cultural resources that people use to resist illness. Such resources might include constitutional strengths (e.g., no history of family illness), social support (e.g., social contacts and social status), and personality dispositions (Kobasa, Maddi, & Kahn, 1982).

Along the lines of resiliency research, Positive Psychology focuses on helping patients achieve positive mood states, instead of simply easing the negative mood state, and thus aims at increasing patients' QoL. Likewise, building positive beliefs, such as optimism, self-esteem, SWB, courage, and the capacity for pleasure and humour, will serve as a protective buffer to ensure future mental health (Seligman, 2002).

In 1987, Antonovsky coined the term "Sense of Coherence" as a protective factor, which decreases psychological distress in the face of adversity. A sense of coherence is experienced when people believe that events are (1) comprehensible (Beliefs: "Life is structured, predictable and explainable.", "It makes sense to me."), (2) manageable (Beliefs: "Personal and external resources are available.", "I have what it takes to do this."), and (3) meaningful (Beliefs: "It fits with my sense of self.", "It's worth it!").

Perceived social support is another known protective factor. Studies have shown that the stronger the perceived social support, the smaller the risk of developing PTSD (e.g., Maercker, 1998). Perceived social support can influence mental and physical health in two ways: firstly, perceived social support can directly lead to greater well-being (main effect), and secondly, it can modify the effect of stressors on well-being (buffer effect). People who have adequate perceived social support believe that they have access to a larger number of coping skills (Lazarus & Folkman, 1984).

Finally, certain coping strategies were found to act as protective factors against psychological distress. Emotion-focused coping and distancing behavior, however, have been found to increase traumatic stress in Western, individualistic cultures (Solomon, Mikulincer, & Avitzur, 1988). Nevertheless, individuals from collectivistic cultures choose these coping strategies more frequently, for example, because compromise and accommodation are regarded as an indication of maturity and tactfulness (Chun, Moos, & Cronkite, 2006). Moreover, denial and avoidance coping were found to decrease traumatic stress in collectivistic cultures (Chang, 2001; Yoshihama, 2002; von Lieres, 2013).

The question arises, how much mental well-being are members of vulnerable groups experiencing, in spite of their hardships? What are the factors that enable them to achieve a sense of psychological well-being? What are their sources of happiness? Which factors protect them from psychological distress? How do they cope with stressful life situations and traumatic events?

The author has tried to answer these questions for an Eastern, collectivistic culture, viz. rural India. The term "collectivistic" was first mentioned by Triandis (1989) in cross-cultural research. In more individualistically-oriented cultures, the self is the central unit of society and individual rights, personal autonomy, and self-fulfilment are emphasised. On the contrary, in more collectivistic-oriented cultures, the in-group forms the central unit of society and duty towards the in-group, interdependence on other group members, and the fulfilment of social roles are emphasised (Hofstede, 1980). It is generally assumed that people from collectivistic cultures have lower QoL and SWB than people from individualistic cultures. However, this could be related to the fact that in collectivistic societies, there is greater pressure to maintain the well-being of the in-group, sometimes at the expense of the individual's well-being (Chun et al., 2006).

How an individual will experience well-being is different for different individuals and cultural groups. Thus, when researchers measure QoL, they need to find out what adds worth to people's lives. It should be the goal of NGOs and other community development agencies to foster the things that are already enhancing the quality of people's lives. Plus, they should take action to mitigate factors currently lowering QoL (Schalock et al., 2002).

## 3 Methods for Sample 1: Tsunami Victims in Kerala, South India

### 3.1 Sample

The sample consisted of 407 inhabitants of the fishing villages along the coastline of Alappad, Kerala. Of these, 233 were affected by the 2004 Asian tsunami and 174 were (comparably) not affected. Respondents affected by the tsunami were in one location where the rise of the ocean had swept away many houses, even though the tsunami did not appear like a tidal wave, as was the case in Tamil Nadu, on the East coast of India. Respondents in the "not affected" group were living near the affected group, but because of a dam, there was no rise of the ocean and no destruction of property. In this way, the total sample was homogeneous regarding socio-economic and demographic factors.

## 3.2 Measurement Tools

A battery of questionnaires was given to the respondents by going from house to house in the two locations in Kollam District along the coastline of Kerala. The items were translated from English into Malayalam and back-translated for accuracy. Since Kerala has the highest literacy rate in all of India, the respondents were able to fill out the questionnaires themselves. A local translator helped to clarify any difficulties in understanding the wording of the items. The level of traumatic stress was measured with the Impact of Event Scale-Revised (IES-R) (Weiss & Marmar, 1996) and general psychological distress with the Brief Symptom Inventory (BSI) (Derogatis, 1993). For measuring the sense of coherence, the Sense of Coherence (SOC) scale was used (Antonovsky, 1987). Different coping strategies were measured with the Brief COPE scale (Carver, 1997). Finally, perceived social support was measured with the Social Support Questionnaire (SOZU-K-22) (Sommer & Fydrich, 1989).

# 4 Results for Sample 1: Tsunami Victims in Kerala, South India

Factor analyzes with the five scales were performed to determine subscales for each scale and to determine whether the originally intended factor-structure of scales could be replicated. Factor analysis with the IES-R led to a two-factor solution: intrusion ($\alpha$ = 0.94) and avoidance ($\alpha$ = 0.87), which corresponds to the factor-structure postulated by the original authors of the IES (Horowitz, Wilner, & Alvarez, 1979). The Brief COPE scale also revealed a two-factor solution: approach coping ($\alpha$ = 0.91) and avoidance coping ($\alpha$ = 0.81). The first factor comprises Folkman and Lazarus' (1980) "problem-focused", as well as "emotion-focused" coping strategies, whereas avoidance coping includes distancing behavior and denial. Factor analyzes with the other scales revealed different factor-structures than intended by the original authors.

To investigate the relationship between psychological distress and protective factors, Pearson's product moment correlations were used. For the tsunami-affected group, a highly significant negative correlation ($p$ < .001) was found between SOC and BSI ($r$ = -0.59**). Perceived social support was negatively correlated with both IES ($r$ = -0.16*) and BSI ($r$ = -0.24**), which means that the higher the perceived social support, the less the extent of traumatisation or any other psychiatric symptoms. Both coping strategies were significantly positively correlated with both variables of traumatic stress.

Linear regression analyzes lead to the following results: In the tsunami-affected group, approach coping significantly predicted a higher IES score ($\beta$ = 0.28**), whereas avoidance-coping did not significantly predict a higher IES score ($\beta = 0.09$). In the total group, approach-coping significantly predicted higher IES scores with beta being $0.30^{**}$ and avoidance-coping significantly predicted lower IES scores with beta being $-0.23^{**}$, which supports the assumption that avoidance-coping is more effective in reducing PTSD in a collectivistic cultural setting. For the BSI, approach-coping also significantly predicted higher scores with beta being $0.17^{**}$. However, avoidance-coping did not predict lower BSI scores significantly.

In a stepwise multiple regression model, the variables SOC, approach-coping, and social support were found to be significant in predicting the BSI score. The standardised beta coefficients were -0.49 for SOC, 0.26 for approach coping, and -0.19 for social support. All three beta coefficients were significant with $p < .001$. SOC, approach coping, and social support together predicted 31.9 % of the variance of the BSI score.

## 5 Discussion for Sample 1: Tsunami Victims in Kerala, South India

Perceived social support, in particular, decreased the level of traumatic stress, and a strong sense of coherence mitigated psychological distress. In the tsunami-affected group, both coping styles were significantly positively correlated with IES-R as well as BSI scores. However, correlations do not give information about causality, and this last finding could also indicate that the more people suffered from symptoms of traumatic stress, the more they engaged in coping efforts. In the total group, however, approach coping increased the level of traumatic stress and avoidance coping reduced it. Therefore, the assumption that avoidance coping is the more effective coping strategy in non-Western, collectivistic cultures, was confirmed.

Implications for practice are that after a natural disaster, protective factors such as perceived social support should be fostered. It is, for example, important that the community support network is not disrupted. Moreover, Western concepts of what effective coping is cannot always be applied in non-Western settings. Therefore, indigenous coping strategies need to be explored and encouraged. For future research, the author suggests that qualitative studies be conducted to explore these coping strategies. Moreover, qualitative studies could explore indigenous ways of experiencing PTSD. To investigate causal relationships, longitudinal studies would be more adequate. In order to generalise the results, similar studies with other indigenous, non-Western samples would be needed.

## 6 Methods for Sample 2: The Rural Population of North India

In 2015, the author conducted a qualitative, exploratory study with residents of villages adopted by Amrita SeRVe in six states of Northern India. The study aimed to explore protective factors for this vulnerable population group. Moreover, the objective was to find out to what extent the village people were satisfied with their lives in spite of adversity.

## 6.1 Focus Group Discussions

Seven focus group discussions were conducted with residents from six villages adopted by Amrita SeRVe. The villages were from six states in North India: Chhattisgarh, Gujarat, Himachal Pradesh, West Bengal, Haryana, and Uttar Pradesh. Each focus group consisted of 4 to 9 informants. Two focus groups were comprised of ladies and five of gents. Men and women were interviewed separately since experience had shown that the village women would not talk freely in the presence of the men. The focus group discussions were facilitated by the author and an interpreter, who translated the author's questions and the informants' responses from Hindi into English.

## 6.2 Qualitative Data Analysis

Content analysis of the transcription texts was conducted to find categories or themes. First, the smallest meaning units were coded to find subcategories, before overall themes or categories of sources of happiness could be found.

# 7 Results for Sample 2: Rural Population of North India

When the informants were asked about whether they were satisfied with their lives, they gave varied responses (see Table 1). It shows that village people are indeed a vulnerable group, as 39% stated that life was difficult and not satisfactory.

"*I am satisfied, but I feel bad about the landless people of my village who have little to support them. They work as unskilled labourers to survive.*"
"*Nobody is satisfied with their life. They always feel, 'I wanted to be this... I wanted to be that.*'"
"*There are five members in my family. I am the only earning member. I work as a farming labourer. We are totally dependent on farming. If there is crop in the fields, we will have food to eat otherwise we have nothing to survive on.*"

Altogether, the informants mentioned more problems than positive aspects of their lives in the villages. Table 2 gives an overview of the frequency and types of problems mentioned.

**Table 1.** Categories and frequencies of different responses about life satisfaction

| 22% | 26% | 13% | 39% |
|---|---|---|---|
| "Life is good/fine." | "Life is OK." | "Life is neither good nor too bad." | "Life is difficult and not satisfactory." |

Table 2. Difficulties mentioned by informants

| Type of Difficulty | Frequency of being mentioned (in % of total statements mentioning difficulties) |
|---|---|
| Poverty | 14 |
| No access to safe drinking water | 11 |
| Health problems | 10 |
| Limited access to quality and higher education | 9 |
| Limited access to medical facilities | 9 |
| No all-weather road | 8 |
| Food insecurity | 8 |
| Drought | 6 |
| Lack of job opportunities | 5 |
| Substance abuse | 5 |
| Low crop yields | 4 |
| No sanitation facilities | 3 |
| Domestic problems | 3 |
| High rate of illiteracy | 3 |
| Limited access to electricity | 2 |

However, with only a few exceptions, all informants stated that they thought it felt better to live in a village than in a city. They believed the village people were happier than city people because of the greenery, beautiful surroundings, fresh air, clean environment, and less stressful life in villages. Further, they believed that village people were more prone to help one another out in times of need and that there was more of a sense of mutual corporation and sense of togetherness.

> "The people in villages are poor, but they greet and respect everyone, whereas in cities, people have a lot of money, but they don't care about their fellow beings. [...] If we see our guest in the village, we will take them to our home. But in cities, if you come across someone, they will ignore you. This is true."
> 
> "There are all the family members and relatives together in the village. There is everything there. So, we feel good there. On the other hand, there is no one in the city whom we can call our own."

We can assume that social support is perceived to a large extent and that this would be a protective factor against psychological distress. Life seems to entail much insecurity regarding the future, especially regarding children's education, income, health care, availability of sufficient food and other basic needs. They mentioned worrying and mental tension.

Table 3. Sources of happiness

| Category | Frequency of being mentioned (in % of total statements mentioning happiness/life satisfaction) |
|---|---|
| Material wealth | 18 |
| Education | 9 |
| Family | 9 |
| Religious/spiritual practices | 8 |
| Work | 8 |
| Serving others | 8 |
| Acceptance | 6 |
| Social support | 5 |
| Having basic needs met | 5 |
| Good health | 5 |
| Studying | 3 |
| Access to medical facilities | 3 |
| Amma's or God's blessings | 2 |
| Being obedient to parents | 1 |

"We have no work, no employment. So how will we say, 'I am good, I am well'?"
"I am concerned about the education of children."
"The children suffer from medical problems, and that is worrying."
"We feel anxious only when we have some problem. [...] Shortage of water is the primary cause of tension. On an average, we feel tense for 3–4 days a week."

In summary, there is the problem of mental tension and worrying about the future among village people. However, the exact scope needs to be explored in further studies. Substance abuse also seems to be a problem in the villages. Likewise, the extent of the problem needs further investigation.

However, in spite of all the hardships of village life, village people seem to be quite happy. Field notes and reports from student interns visiting the villages have revealed that villagers were frequently smiling and seemed to be happy. One lady from Himachal summed up the mental state of the villagers accordingly: *"Sometimes we do feel upset, but generally we are happy."*

When the informants were asked to name sources of happiness, or "what made them happy" or "who is a happy person", the following categories emerged (see table 3):

## 8 Discussion for Sample 2: Rural Populations in North India

India's rural areas are the ones least benefitting from India's growing GDP and generally do not experience economic prosperity. For them, life is still a struggle for survival. Therefore, a large percentage of sources of happiness mentioned by the informants related to material wealth, such as having a high income or owning a big house or car. They need money to meet their most basic needs, so money is seen as a source of happiness. Education is also very important, as having education will help villagers hold a better-paid job. Nevertheless, not all informants agreed that money makes people happy. Some said that poor people could also be happy. Accepting one's circumstances and adjusting to what one has was also viewed as a viable source of happiness. Still, the most basic needs of having a roof over one's head and enough food to eat should be met to be happy. Further, there should be access to health care, since a healthy body is a prerequisite for a happy life.

Moreover, in close-knit, collectivistic communities, the well-being of the group is considered more important than the feelings and beliefs of the individual (Triandis, 1989). In line with living in a collectivistic society, living with family members, receiving social support, but also obeying parents was considered necessary for happiness. Simply having a family and living with parents and children was seen as more important than having loving relationships within the family. Many informants stated that they derived much happiness from doing their daily work, e.g. farming work. Performing religious or spiritual practices, such as praying or surrendering everything to God's will, as well as serving others, was also mentioned quite frequently as a source of happiness. All these sources of happiness can be seen as protective factors, which help village people endure hardships and insecurity regarding the future.

## 9 Conclusion

In conclusion, much work still needs to be done by Amrita SeRVe and other organizations to eliminate abject poverty and to transform the lives of vulnerable populations, whether they are survivors of disasters or not. It is crucial to let the voices of marginalised groups be heard and to find out which resources are available to them to serve as protective factors. We should then give priority to strengthening those factors. Future research will show how to do this.

In both samples, perceived social support emerges as a crucial protective factor. This has implications for future disaster aid projects: extended families need to be housed together, and social support networks maintained. Communities need to be shifted as a whole to a new location if evacuation becomes necessary. Further, activities can be performed to strengthen a sense of unity, for example, sports events, games for the children, teaching vocational skills to groups of women, etc.

## 10 Affiliation

Dr. Johanna Sophie von Lieres
Institution: Center for Women's Empowerment and Gender Equality, Amrita Vishwa Vidyapeetham, Amritapuri, India
Address: Clappana, Kollam District, Kerala, India
E-mail: sophia.vonlieres@ammachilabs.org

## 11 References

Antonovsky, A. (1979). *Health, stress and coping.* San Francisco, CA: Jossey-Bass.

Antonovsky, A. (1987). *Unravelling the mystery of health. How people manage stress and stay well.* San Francisco, CA: Jossey-Bass.

Becker, G. S., Philipson, T. J., & Soares, R. R. (2003). *The quantity and quality of life and the evolution of world inequality. NBER Working Paper No. 9765.* Cambridge, MA: National Bureau of Economic Research.

Carver, C.S. (1997). You want to measure coping but your protocol is too long: Consider the Brief COPE. *International Journal of Behavioral Medicine, 4,* 92–100.

Census of India. (2011). *Census of India 2011. Rural urban distribution of population (Provisional population totals).* Retrieved on May 31, 2012 from http://censusindia.gov.in/2011-prov-results/paper2/data_files/india/Rural_Urban_2011.pdf

Chang, E. C. (2001). A look at the coping strategies and styles of Asian Americans: Similar and different? In C. R. Snyder (Ed.), *Coping with stress: Effective people and processes,* 222–239. London: Oxford University Press.

Chun, C.-A., Moos, R. H., & Cronkite, R. C. (2006). Culture: A fundamental context for the stress and coping paradigm. In P. T. P. Wong & L. C. J. Wong (Eds.), *Handbook of multicultural perspectives on stress and coping,* 29–53. New York: Springer.

Derogatis, L. R. (1993). *Brief symptom inventory (BSI), administration, scoring, and procedures manual* (3rd ed.). Minneapolis: National Computer Services.

Diener, E. (1984). Subjective well-being. *Psychological Bulletin, 95*(3), 542–575.

Diener, E., Diener, M., & Diener, C. (1995). Factors predicting the subjective well-being of nations. *Journal of Personality and Social Psychology, 69*(5), 851–864.

Folkman, S., & Lazarus, R. S. (1980). An analysis of coping in a middle-aged community sample. *Journal of Health & Social Behavior, 21,* 219–239.

Goel, D. S., Agarwal, S. P., Ichhpujani, R. L., & Shrivastana, S. (2004). Chapter 1. Mental health in 2003: The Indian scene. In S. P. Agarwaal, D. S. Goel, R. L. Ichhpujani, R. N. Salhan, & S. Shrivatsava (Eds.), *Mental Health – An Indian perspective (1946–2003)*, (pp. 3–24). New Delhi: Directorate General of Health Services, Ministry of Health and Family Welfare.

Hofstede, G. (1980). *Culture's consequences: Comparing values, behaviors, institutions and organizations across nations.* Beverly Hills, CA: Sage.

Horowitz, M. J., Wilner, N., & Alvarez, W. (1979). Impact of Event Scale: A measure of subjective stress. *Psychosomatic Medicine, 41*(3), 209–218.

Kobasa, S. C., Maddi, S. R., & Kahn, S. (1982). Hardiness and health: A prospective study. *Journal of Personality and Social Psychology, 42* (1), 168–177s.

Lazarus, R. S., & Folkman, S. (1984). *Stress, appraisal, and coping.* New York: Springer.

Maercker, A. (1998). *Posttraumatische Belastungsstörungen: Psychologie der Extrembelastungsfolgen bei Opfern politischer Gewalt.* Lengerich: Pabst.

Mukunthan, A. (2015). Rural India is far behind urban India in every indicator of progress. *Factly, December 5, 2015.* Retrieved on February 4, 2018 from https://factly.in/rural-india-behind-urban-india-in-progress-indicators/

Schalock, R. L., Brown, I., Brown, R., Cummins, R. A., Felce, D., Matikka, L., ..., & Parmenter, T. (2002). Conceptualization, measurement, and application of quality of life for persons with intellectual disabilities: Report of an international panel of experts. *Mental Retardation, 40*(6), 457–470s.

Seligman, M. (2002). *Authentic happiness. Using the new positive psychology to realize your potential for lasting fulfilment.* Boston, MA: Nicholas Brealey.

Socio-Economic Census. (2011). *I- Key findings from rural India.* Retrieved from http://www.secc.gov.in/reportlistContent

Solomon, Z., Mikulincer, M., & Avitzur, E. (1988). Coping, locus of control, social support, and combat-related post-traumatic stress disorder – a prospective study. *Journal of Personality and Social Psychology, 55,* 279–285.

Sommer, G., & Fydrich, T. (1989). *F-SOZU. Fragebogen zur Sozialen Unterstützung. Soziale Unterstützung, Diagnostik, Konzepte, F-SOZU* (DGVT Materiale Nr. 22). Tuebingen: Deutsche Gesellschaft für Verhaltenstherapie.

Triandis, H. C. (1989). The self and social behaviour in differing cultural contexts. *Psychological Review, 96*(3), 506–520.

von Lieres, J. S. (2013). Tsunami in Kerala, India: Long-term psychological distress, sense of coherence, and coping in a non-industrialized setting. In E. Witruk (Ed.), *Beiträge zur Pädagogischen und Rehabilitationspsychologie, Band 5.* Frankfurt am Main: Peter Lang.

Weiss, D. S., & Marmar, C. R. (1996). The Impact of Event Scale-Revised. In J. P. Wilson & T. M. Keane (Eds.), *Assessing psychological trauma and PTSD,* 399–411. New York: Guilford.

World Health Organization Regional Office for South-East Asia. (2005). WHO framework for mental health and psychosocial support after the tsunami.

Retrieved on May 19, 2012 from http://www.searo.who.int/entity/emergencies/documents/sea_earthquake_and_tsunami_framework.pdf?ua=1

Yoshihama, M. (2002). Battered women's coping strategies and psychological distress: Differences by immigration status. *American Journal of Community Psychology, 30*(3), 429–452.

Asanka Bulathwatta and Evelin Witruk

# Trauma and Coping Styles among University Students in Sri Lanka and Germany: Role of Emotional Intelligence and Resilience

**Abstract:** Individual coping is a discussion in the domain of stress, daily hazards and some interpersonal domains. Trauma coping considered to be a complex phenomenon rather simply mean of stress coping strategies because traumatic events and traumas considered to be a factor effect on our cognition. These coping strategies can be approached as well as avoidance of the occurred traumatic event. The main objective of this study was to identify the role of Emotional Intelligence in developing coping strategies among people who faced traumatic events and controlling the effect of resilience. Subjects of this study were 356 university students from Germany and Sri Lanka. Bivariate correlations, hierarchical multiple regression analysis, regression analysis with mediation and path models were performed to test the hypotheses. The results revealed that the German and Sri Lankan students show a different level of Emotional Intelligence and its influencing different way of determining coping strategies. German student's resilience capacity show significantly negative correlation with the Emotional intelligence. The current study indicated the direct and indirect effect of Trauma symptoms. It shows some significant difference between German and Sri Lankan students. Level of exposure to traumatic events also indicated differently in between two countries. Surprisingly human-made trauma is a common phenomenon in both countries. Coping styles from both countries show significance difference.

**Keywords:** emotional intelligence, resilience, trauma, coping

## 1 Introduction

This study tried to figure out the role of Emotional Intelligence (EI) for developing coping strategies among adolescents who face traumatic events. Late adolescence students who have enrolled in the university education (e.g., Bachelors/Masters) were selected as the sample. University education is an important stage of students' academic life. Therefore, all students need to develop their competencies to attain the goal of passing examinations and also to develop their wisdom related to the scientific knowledge they gathered through their academic life. A study has been conducted in a cross-cultural manner, and it took place in Germany and Sri Lanka. Late adolescence is a critical period of the human being as it is a stage in life which acquiring the emotional and social qualities of social life. There are many adolescents who have affected by traumatic events during their lifespan but have not been identified or treated. More specifically, there are numerous burning issues within the first year of the university students, namely ragging that done by seniors to juniors, bullying, invalidation, and issues raise based on attitudes changes and orientation issues. Those factors can be traumatic for both academic and day to day lifestyle. Older, involved in ragging students sometimes have to left the university (as a result of suspension). Younger students may be traumatised as victims of Ragging and thus impaired their social life. Determining the resilience, emotional damage, post-traumatic stress disorder of those affected by ragging are strictly necessary to achieve effective rehabilitation of students regarding their academic performance of their social life at the university.

Emotional involvement in trauma is not vastly studied in the field of Trauma Psychology. Therefore, identifying the emotional background for the context of trauma coping is an immensely needed precondition. The general question of this study is to explore how emotional capacity (i.e., Emotional Intelligence) and recovery capacity (i.e., resilience) can influence coping processes after the traumatic experience of university students. The cross-cultural format of the study was chosen to compare samples with expected low and high traumatic experiences in two different cultural contexts and the way react with their emotional and recovery capacities to develop coping through the trauma.

The main focus of the current study is to find out the role of EI in developing coping strategies among people who faced traumatic events and controlling the effect of resilience.

## 2 Theoretical Review

Germany and Sri Lanka are two different countries not only in terms of the location, development status in the world, but also the cultural components. According to The Hofstede Center (2015), Sri Lanka is a highly collectivistic country, meanwhile, Germany is individualistic. Therefore, this different cultural background influences on all social and cultural phenomenon likewise also the processes of traumatic experiences.

Trauma is an overall existing presence, and it is represented by war, natural disasters, and individual trauma. Diagnostic and Statistical Manual of Mental Disorders fifth edition (DSM-V) defines a trauma or a traumatic event as an experience that causes physical, emotional and psychological distress or harm (American Psychiatric Association, 2013). Moreover, DSM-V points out that there are different types of traumatic events, namely natural disasters (i.e., hurricane, flood, tornado), industrial disasters, accidents (i.e., car and train), childhood sexual abuse, rape, criminal victimisation, and domestic violence (American Psychiatric Association, 2013).

Trauma can be varied according to the context it happened. Type I trauma refers to the single unexpected direct traumas in our life. Type II trauma refers to ongoing chronic traumatic conditions (e.g., poverty, hunger illnesses, physical and sexual abuse) and past extended traumatic conditions to the present time. Type III traumas refer to the traumas can be affected in one area of human functions, e.g., attachment or survival or it can affect different or all areas of individual processing (Kira, 2001).

Most of the victims who are affected by traumatic events show many emotional disturbances and damages resulting in drastic life changes. Among the most prevalent symptoms of traumatic events are behavioral and mood changes, such as sleeplessness, loss of appetite, and emptiness of facial expressions. However, the underlying emotions that cause the superficial reactions that can be observed are not easily revealed.

Therefore, it is essential to understand the emotions of the affected persons and their EI to help them with a reliable coping strategy (Bulathwatta, 2013).

# 3 Method

## 3.1 Sample

The samples in this study consist of 356 university students from Germany and Sri Lanka. There are 149 German students who studied in the University of Leipzig, Germany in two different faculties (Institute of Psychology and Faculty of Education) and 207 Sri Lankan students from the Department of Philosophy and Psychology in the University of Peradeniya and in the Department of Educational Psychology, Faculty of Education in the University of Colombo. There were 11.8% males and 88.2% female participants represented the sample. Those who were coming from different stages of their university life: 60.1% were bachelor students, 1.7% were master students, and 37.6% were represented the Educational degree. The majority of students were in the aged between 19 to 24 Years.

## 3.2 Measurement Tools

### 3.2.1 Questionnaire

Identification of the dimensions of EI will be measured with Trait Emotional Intelligence Questionnaire (TEI-Que; Cooper & Petrides, 2010; Petrides & Furnham, 2006) while coping strategies are measured with Brief Coping Inventory (Carver, 1997). Students' resilience capacity which means the one's ability to adapt to stressful or crisis situations will be measured with the Resilience Scale for Children and Adolescents (Emotional Reactivity Scale; Prince-Embury, 2006. Effects of traumatic events faced by the students are identified with the Essener Trauma Inventory (Tagay & Senf, 2009). Traumatic events which affected the university students from their childhood will be measured with the Childhood Trauma Questionnaire (CTQ; Bernstein & Fink, 1998).

Theoretically, following causal model (Figure 1) is showing the relationships between the main constructs emotional intelligence, resilience, trauma symptoms, approach and avoidance coping derived.

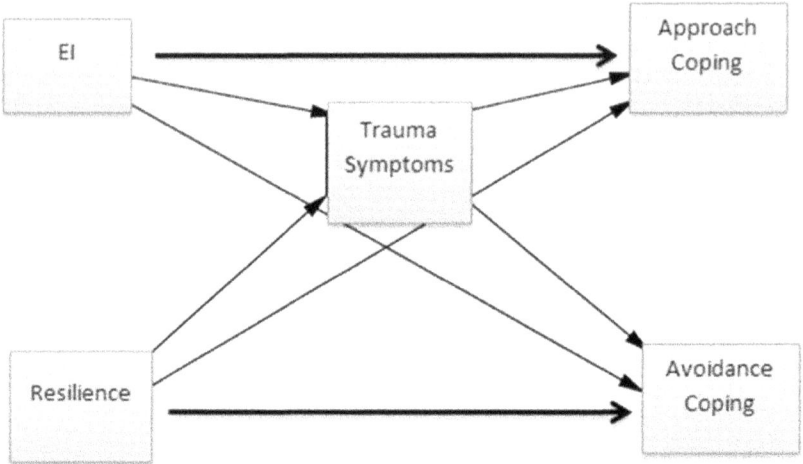

**Figure 1.** Causal model of relationship of predictors and outcome and mediator

## 4 Results

Bivariate correlation, hierarchical multiple regression analysis, mediation analysis with regression, and path model were performed in order to test the hypothesis considered in the research. The current study was based upon fifteen hypotheses which testing results here will be reported by examples.

Level of EI in between German students and Sri Lankan students show a significant difference; German students tend to use EI was significantly lower than the Sri Lankan students level of using EI ($\beta = -0.23$, $p < 0.001$).

Meanwhile, the resilience capacity that was measured through the sense of mastery and emotional reactions among German students showed statistically lower than the Sri Lankan students ($\beta = 0.37$, $p < 0.01$), but the emotional reaction capacity among German students is statistically higher than the Sri Lankan students ($\beta = -0.22$, $p < 0.001$).

Results indicate that significantly German students use more approach coping when they overcoming traumatic experiences than the Sri Lankan students. Even though German students statistically show lower EI than the Sri Lankan students, but this variable was a significant predictor for approach coping among German students ($\beta = 0.05$, $p < 0.001$). However, statistically, the EI among Sri Lankan students was not a significant predictor of their approach coping style. Whereas emotional reactions and sense of mastery play significant roles in this sense ($\beta = -0.22$, $p < 0.001$). Considering the avoidance coping styles of the German students, EI was not a significant predictor to determine the style. However, Sri Lankan students use their EI to react using avoidance coping styles ($\beta = -0.13$, $p$

< 0.001). Resilience also plays a significant role in this sense among Sri Lankan students ($\beta$ = -0.05, $p$ < 0.001).

Considering the mediation role of the traumatic symptoms (i.e., dissociation, avoidance, hyper arousal, and intrusion) within EI and approach coping style, the mediation effect was indicated only within Sri Lankan students. The process is the same about the sense of avoidance coping, which emerged only among Sri Lankan students. Surprisingly, the mediation effect between trauma symptoms within resilience and approach coping style emerge only with Sri Lankan students. Last but not least, the results indicated that the mediation effect of trauma symptoms between resilience and avoidance coping style only appear among the Sri Lankan students.

## 5 Conclusion

Results of the current study indicate that German and Sri Lankan students show two different patterns in terms of trauma coping and the role of their EI and resilience. German students used a lower level of EI than the Sri Lankan students when they overcome trauma. Sri Lankan students were in the opposite side from them. More specifically, German students tend to use their emotional reaction capacity as a part of resilience within traumas, whereas Sri Lankan students used their sense of mastery skills as a part of resilience during the process of developing coping style within traumas. It leads to the assumption that German students are strong in emotional reaction ability, whereas Sri Lankan students are strong in developing a sense of mastery of their traumatic events. Mediation effect of trauma symptoms also indicated a specific condition within two different students sample as a representation of two different cultural backgrounds.

The current study has certain limitations, such as the study could measure only a part of the real complexity of the phenomenon. There was a lack of previous studies connected to the EI and coping style with trauma. The two samples showed significant similarities regarding sex ratio (more female participants) and based on the selected disciplines (especially Psychology and disciplines related to Psychology).

Trauma is a never-ending phenomenon in the modern and rapidly changing world. The students were confronted with few natural and more personal trauma in their lifetime. Some will be further affected in their lives by these traumatic burdens. Psychological student counselling and better career guidance at the university would be strongly recommended to find a solution to these problems.

## 6 Affiliations

Dr. Asanka Bulathwatta
Institution/address: Department of Psychology, Faculty of Arts, University of Peradeniya, Peradeniya, 20400, Sri Lanka.
E-mail: asankabulathwatta@gmail.com

Prof. Dr. Evelin Witruk
Institution: Institute of Psychology, University of Leipzig, Germany
Address: Neumarkt 9-19, 04109 Leipzig, Germany
E-mail: witruk@uni-leipzig.de

# 7 References

American Psychiatric Association (Ed.). (2013). Diagnostic and Statistical Manual of Mental Disorders: DSM-5 (5th). Washington, D.C.: American Psychiatric Association.

American Psychiatric Association. (2013). *Diagnostic and statistical manual of mental disorders* (5th ed.). Washington, DC

Bernstein, D. P, & Fink, L. (1998). *Childhood Trauma Questionnaire: A retrospective self-report manual.* San Antonio, TX: The Psychological Corporation.

Bulathwatta, A. (2013). Trauma and Coping among University students. Exploring Emotional Intelligence Application on Coping with Trauma. *Arbeitstitle-Forum für Leipziger Promovirende, 2*(5), 29–35. Retrieved on February 20, 2018 from http://www.wissens-werk.de/index.php/arbeitstitel/article/viewFile/159/215

Carver, C. S. (1997). You want to measure coping but your protocol's too long: consider the briefCOPE. *International Journal of Behavioral Medicine, 4*(1), 92–100. doi:10.1207/s15327558ijbm0401_6

Cooper, A. & Petrides, K. V. (2010). A psychometric analysis of the Trait Emotional Intelligence Questionnaire-Short Form (TEIQue-SF) using Item Response Theory. *Journal of Personality Assessment, 92,* 449–457.

Kira, I. A. (2001). Taxonomy of trauma and trauma assessment. *Traumatology, 7*(2), 73–86. doi:10.1177/153476560100700202

Petrides, K. V., & Furnham, A. (2006). The Role of Trait Emotional Intelligence in a Gender-Specific Model of Organizational Variables. *Journal of Applied Social Psychology, 36,* 552–569.

Prince-Embury, S. (2006). *Resiliency Scales for children and adolescents: A profile of personal strengths* (1st ed.). San Antonio, TX: Harcourt Assessment. Retrieved on March 3, 2012 from http://www.PsychCorp.com

Tagay, S., & Senf, W. (2009). Essener Trauma – Inventer, Fremdbeurteilung. Essen: LVR-Klinikum Essen, Universitaet Duisburg.

The Hofstede Center. (2015). Sri Lanka and Germany Comparison of cultural dimensions. Retrieved on November 5, 2016 from http://geert-hofstede.com/sri_lanka.html

Nadia Hanum
# Trauma after Accident: Case Study of Traffic Accident Survivors with Spinal Cord Injury in Indonesia

**Abstract:** Surviving from an accident or become witnesses of the accident was a terrible experience for everyone. Bad memories about the accident, the feeling that cannot receive physical disability after the accident, and avoiding feeling to go back again to drive are overshadowing the victims after discharged from the hospital. Four patients in an Orthopaedic Hospital in Surakarta, Indonesia were interviewed from first month after their accident. The aim of this study is to analyze the development of the psychological condition of the traffic accidents victims with spinal cord from the time the initial reaction of shock to trauma. Physical paralyzed in the lower part of the body develops anxiety, withdrawing from others, irritability, denial, and hopeless. This condition can be categorized as a reaction of shock after traffic accident and can lead to trauma. Several aspects have been explored in the interview, namely cognitive or belief, culture, educational background and social status. The results suggest the need for early screening of trauma after the accident to optimize for recovery and rehabilitation.

**Keywords:** trauma, traffic accident, traffic and transportation psychology

## 1 Introduction

Motor vehicle crashes (MVCs) are a major cause of death and disability worldwide (Joseph et al., 2014). As many other countries may recognize that there are three main causes of traffic accidents, namely, human factors, vehicle factors, and road and environmental factors, Indonesia also has there. It is, however, true that non-human factors in Indonesia have a greater percentage as compared to other countries, figures, and implicitly indicate human errors too, such as ignorance of human to vehicle and road maintenance (Soehodho, 2009).

Several studies have shown that traffic accidents are a common cause of post-traumatic stress disorder (PTSD). Ursano et al. (1999) and Bryant, Marozzeky, Crooks, Gurka (2004) found a prevalence of 25% PTSD three months and 18% six months after the traffic accident. PTSD seems to be an important psychological consequence of accidents with motorized vehicles. Most studies involve populations of patients selected according to the kind of injury caused by the accident, e.g., an orthopedic trauma (Starr et al., 2004), a spinal cord trauma (Nielsen, 2003) or a brain trauma (Harvey & Bryant, 2000).

Ursano et al. (1999) also reported that a previous trauma does not seem to be a risk factor, although a previous episode of PTSD does. Richmond and Kauder

(2000) identified four variables that were important in the prediction of psychological distress after a serious injury, namely increased levels of psychological distress during hospitalization, a positive screen for drugs and alcohol at the time of the injury, young age, and the lack of anticipation of possible problems that can occur with when resuming normal activities.

## 2 Theoretical Review

Accidents are the most common civilian trauma. Through their unpredictability, suddenness, uncontrollability and danger to life, health and integrity they have a high potential of trauma. In a subset it comes to the chronicity of the initial shock, stress, and stress reactions. Unfavourable healing processes, massive suffering of the survivors, family environment as well as high costs of health and social security systems are the consequences (Maercker, 2013).

Trauma seems to be an important psychological consequence of accidents with motorized vehicles. It has prevalence of 25% PTSD three months and 18% six months after the traffic accident (Ursano, 1999) and other researchers noted the prevalence of PTSD following a Motor Vehicle Accident (MVA) range from 1% (Breslau, Davis, Andreski, & Peterson, 1991) to 39% (Blanchard, Hickling, Taylor, & Loos, 1995), with higher rates found in studies that assessed help-seeking samples and lower rates found in more general epidemiological surveys.

Symptoms of PTSD after Accidents are often in various, typical patterns. Turnbull (1999) described the main clusters of PTSD from the MVA perspective. The symptoms for PTSD fall into three categories, intrusion (in people with PTSD, memories of the trauma reoccur unexpectedly, episodes called "flashbacks" intrude into their current lives, and flashback of accidents), avoidance (avoidance symptoms – avoidance and fear in traffic, no return to drive and no back to the road), and hyper arousal (concentration and attentional deficits, and hyper vigilance).

## 3 Method

### 3.1 Participant

The participants of this study were four MVA survivors who got an accident more than a year and suffered currently from severe injury. All of them suffered spinal cord injury and paralyzed.

### 3.2 Measurement Tools

This study will be carried out as a qualitative method using case study research design. It means the qualitative interview technique will be used and the assessment takes place only with a small sample. For this reason, the author will use different clinical interview techniques of this research area:

a. The half standardized interview with aspects to be explored:
1) Cognitive and belief aspect
2) Cultural aspect
3) Personality aspect
4) Family support
5) The effectiveness of medical rehabilitation for mental health and recovery
b. PTSS-10 (Maercker, 1998).

The last interview will be done also with the purpose to classify the subjects as PTSD symptom holders who suffering from PTSD in a severe level. The criteria for PTSD in the PTSS-10 is 12 and will be reached by all subjects.

## 3.3 Analysis

The content analysis procedure was used for this case study analysis. Qualitative content analysis is an approach to documents that emphasizes the role of the investigator in the construction of the meaning of and in texts. There is an emphasis on allowing categories to emerge out of data and on recognizing the significance for understanding the meaning of the context in which an item being analyzed (and the categories derived from it) appeared (Bryman, 2004).

According to Mayring (2003), qualitative content analysis can be divided into nine different stages:

a. determination of the material;
b. analysis of the situation in which the text originated;
c. the formal characterization of the material;
d. determination of the direction of the analysis;
e. theoretically informed differentiation of questions to be answered;
f. selection of the analytical techniques (summary, explication, structuring);
g. definition of the unit of analysis;
h. analysis of the material (summary, explication, structuring); and
i. interpretation.

# 4 Results

The content analyzis under the perspective of cognitions and beliefs shows high evidence with clear and subjective representation of the main symptoms of PTSD after accident of the survivors. The accident experiences and injury consequences were also reported, e.g., statements according to the PTSD-symptom level of the accident (i.e., sleep and eating disorders), disturbed emotionality (i.e., anxiety, other reactive behaviors, and refusing of help), avoidance, and suicidal behavior. One of the most frequent statements was according to the unexpectedness of the accident, to the severe sleep disturbances (including nightmares), to anxiety symptoms and avoidance. The faith of God and forgiveness seems to be specific for the Indonesian's society, which in majority is Muslim. Symptoms are not only from the direct consequence of the body distortions, but also from a spiritual consequence.

It is possible to sort the statements into three general cultural categories concerning different forms of obtained support, such as support from neighbours, friends, and family. It is obvious that friends, family members, and neighbours have different forms of support. In all main categories, typical features of a Muslim society are obvious, for instance related to the money collection, visiting and praying together in the neighbourhood.

The survivors have variety of categories, such as personality traits, coping styles of personality, and personality determined forms of abreactions. The accident is always a hard phase in survivors' life. Nevertheless, the personality described them to have capability to overcome their problems before the last accident happened (resiliency); personality changed after accident (self-description and description by others); and spirituality played a special role in survivors' recovery phase. The future orientation of personality and the mind must always become the positive aspects. Spirituality is hereby as a coping strategy. Whereas believing in God's will help to find the solution of the problems and this is one feature of self-motivation.

During hospital phase of rehabilitation, participants reported the psychological rehabilitation once a week, but in the outpatient phase of rehabilitation, there was no further psychological rehabilitation. Overall, the effectiveness of the rehabilitation system is influenced by the perceived integration of hospital and outpatient phase during the treatment, which are important for the patients. Financial resources play an important role in the extent of given and received treatment in the hospital. Psychological based rehabilitation of drivers after MVA is not common and could not found in all participants. Furthermore, there is a lack of specialists who can deliver psychological help for MVA survivors after the hospital phase.

# 5 Discussion

The numbers of traffic accidents in Indonesia increased year by year. Even though the characteristic of the sample can be categorized as normal drivers, however, still traffic accidents could not be avoided. The absence of post-crash care programs in Indonesia can be one of the factors that may cause psychological trauma among MVA survivors. The hidden fear of the MVA survivors can be seen through the PTSD symptoms and the level of the chronic stress among the survivors, which could be demonstrated in the results of this research. The PTSD symptom that has been showed by most survivors is avoidance coping strategy. The author found a clear evidence that the anxiety of the survivors to start driving again after accident appear, and there is a high level of avoidance behavior to start driving after accident or going back alone in the traffic.

All survivors/participants reported that the last accident was an unexpected event that overwhelms their emotional and physical state. However, the traumatic event is not always only a distressing event. Tedeschi and Calhoun (1996) have noted that traumatic events that confront the individual may become a challenge of how to make the experience manageable, comprehensible, and meaningful. Successful adaptation requires effective negotiation of these psychological tasks, which in turn can provide the base for positive individual and personal changes called posttraumatic growths. The successful adaptation can be improved by the help of psychological intervention during the recovery phase. This intervention can help survivors to overcome and healing the psychological wound after the MVA. It has been clear, that the post-crash care program for MVA survivors is huge necessary, especially for Indonesia. For that reason, the role and impact of traffic psychology and training related to it in the universities and specialist program for psychotherapists must be improved. In the end, the cultural and natural resources of the society in a Muslim country should be considered further.

# 6 Affiliation

Dr. Nadia Hanum
Institution: Department of Clinical Psychology and Psychotherapy, University of Leipzig.
Address: Insitute of Psychology, University of Leipzig, Neumarkt 9–19, 04109 Leipzig, Germany.
E-Mail: dhea_nadia@yahoo.com

# 7 References

Blanchard, E. B., Hickling, E., Taylor, A., & Loos, W. (1995). Psychiatric morbidity associated with motor vehicle accidents. *Journal of Nervous and Mental Disease, 183*, 495–504.

Breslau, N., Davis, G. C., Andreski, P., & Peterson, E. (1991). Traumatic events and posttraumatic stress disorder in an urban population of young adults. *Archives of General Psychiatry, 48*, 216–222.

Bryant, R. A., Marosszeky, J. E., Crooks, J., & Gurka, J. A. (2004). Elevated resting heart rate as a predictor of posttraumatic stress disorder after severe traumatic brain injury. *Psychosomatic Medicine, 66*(5), 760–761.

Bryman, A.lan (2004). *Social research methods* (2nd ed.). New York: Oxford University Press.

Harvey, A. G., & Bryant, R. A. (2000). Two-year prospective evaluation of the relationship between acute stress disorder and posttraumatic stress disorder following mild traumatic brain injury. *American Journal of psychiatry, 157*, 626–628.

Joseph, P. G., Odonnell, M. J., Teo, K. K., Gao, P., Anderson, C., Probstfield, J. L. …Yusuf, S. (2014). The Mini-Mental State Examination, Clinical Factors, and

Motor Vehicle Crash Risk. *Journal of the American Geriatrics Society, 62*(8), 1419–1426. doi:10.1111/jgs.12936

Maercker, A. (1998). Posttraumatische Stress Skala-10 (PTSS-10) – deutsche Version modifiziert nach Schueffel u. Schade. *Klinische Psychologie II*. Zürich: Universität Zürich.

Maercker, A. (2013). *Posttraumatische Belastungsstörungen: Mit 10 Tabellen und zahlreichen Fallbeispielen*. Heidelberg: Springer.

Mayring, P. (2003). *Qualitative Inhaltsanalyse, Grundlagen und Techniken* (8th ed.). Weinheim: Beltz, UTB.

Nielsen, M. S. (2003). Prevalence of posttraumatic stress disorder in persons with spinal cord injuries: The mediating effect of social support. *Rehabilitation Psychology, 48* (4), 289–295.

Richmond, T. S., & Kauder, D. (2000). Predictors of psychological distress following serious injury. *Journal of Traumatic Stress, 13* (4), 681–692.

Soehodho, S. (2009). *Road Accidents in Indonesia*. Director of Center for Transport Studies. Jakarta: University of Indonesia.

Starr, A. J., Smith, W. R., Frawley, W. H., Borer, D. S., Morgan, S. J., Reinert, C. M., & Mendoza-Welch, M. (2004). Symptoms of posttraumatic stress disorder after orthopaedic trauma. *The Journal of Bone and Joint Surgery, 86* (6), 1115–1120.

Tedeschi, R. G., & Calhoun, L. G. (1996). The Posttraumatic Growth Inventory: Measuring the positive legacy of trauma. *Journal of Traumatic Stress, 9*, 455–47.

Turnbull, G. (1999). Survival, Fear, Post-Traumatic Stress Disorder and All That. In *The International Handbook of Road Traffic Accidents & Psychological Trauma: Current Understanding. Treatment and Law* (pp. 15–28). Oxford: Pergamon.

Ursano, R. J., Fullerton, C. S., Epstein, R. S., Crowley, B., Vance, K., Kao, T. C. & Baum, A. (1999). Peritraumatic dissociation and posttraumatic stress disorder following motor vehicle accidents. *American Journal of Psychiatry, 156*, 1808–1810.

# Chapter 2  Stress Experiences

Marcus Stueck, Hans-Ullrich Balzer, Sebastian Mueller,
Dian Sari Utami, & Ulrich Sack

# Das mobile Gesundheitslabor: Ein Bestandteil des Gesundheitswürfels zur Psychischen Gefährdungs- und Ressourcenbeurteilung im Rahmen des Biozentrisch-betrieblichen Gesundheitsmanagements

**Abstract:** The Health Laboratory is a concept which components where developed, in the last years of the 90th during an expedition to the Aconcagua (in Argentina, 6995 m) and several expeditions to the Cho Oyu Mountain (in Tibet, 8206 m) and Pakistan (Gasherbrum 1 and 2 in 1996 and 1997). There the alpinists took a simple measurement tools (e.g., skin response devices HIMEM and questionnaires for estimating their stress states. After the successful measurements in long-term monitoring of the stress behavior, two concepts began to grow in stressful fields: the concept of multilevel psychological diagnostic of psychic risk patterns (Health Cube) with the mobile health laboratory. The chronobiological basics measurement tools were used (i.e., stress-diagnostic test, blood pressure relaxation test) as well as new developments in this fields (skin sensibility) and out of the psycho-neuro-immunological field (Cortisol). In this article the measurement procedures of the Mobile Health Lab are explained and with examples introduced.

**Keywords:** mobile health laboratory, chrono-bio-psychology, stress-diagnostic procedures, health cube, Biocentric Occupational Health Management

**Zusammenfassung:** Das Gesundheitslabor ist ein Konzept, das in den 90er Jahren während verschiedener Hochgebirgsexpeditionen (in Argentinien, 6995 m; in Tibet, 8206 m; in Pakistan, Gasherbrum 1 und 2 in 1996 und 1997) entwickelt wurde. Dort nutzten die Alpinisten einfache Messinstrumente (z. B. Hautreaktionsgeräte HIMEM und Fragebögen zur Abschätzung ihrer Stresszustände). Nach den erfolgreichen Messungen im Langzeitmonitoring wurde das Konzept der multimethodalen psychologischen Diagnostik psychischer Risikomuster (Gesundheitswürfel) mit dem mobilen Gesundheitslabor entwickelt. Hierbei spielen entwickelten chronobiologischen Grundlagen-Messinstrumente eine Rolle (Stressdiagnostischer Test, Blutdruck-Relaxationstest) sowie neue Entwicklungen auf diesem Gebiet (Hautsensibilität) und psychoneuroimmunologische Felddiagnostik (Cortisol). Es werden die Messverfahren des Mobile Health Lab erläutert und mit Beispielen vorgestellt.

**Schlüsselworte:** Mobiles Gesundheitslabor, Chronobiopsychologie, Stress-diagnostische Meßprozeduren, Gesundheitswürfel, Biozentrisches Betriebliches Gesundheitsmanagement

## 1 Einleitende Bemerkungen zum Mobilen Gesundheitslabors

Zur Durchführung einfacher physiologischer Verhaltensparameter wurde seit 2002 an der Universität Leipzig das Konzept eines Mobilen Gesundheitslabors (Balzer & Stueck, 2019) entwickelt und an der DPFA-Hochschule Sachsen in Leipzig weiter ausgebaut. Hier wird es zur Diagnostik aber auch zum Training (*Biofeedback*) in Schulen, Kindertagesstätten, Reha-Kliniken, Gesundheitstagen für das Betriebliche Gesundheitsmanagement genutzt. Es ist Teil des Gesundheitswürfels (Ebene 2; Stueck, 2019), welcher auf 6 Ebenen Analysen zur Psychischen Gefährdungsbeurteilung vornimmt. Das Laborkonzept wurde auch an der Islamischen Universität Yogyakarta in Indonesien bzw. an der Universität Teheran (für Berufskraftfahrer) umgesetzt bzw. aufgebaut. Im Rahmen des Mobilen Gesundheitslabors können mit verschiedenen Zielgruppen (z.B. Lehrer/Erzieher, Pflegeberufe, Hochschulen, Klinikspersonal, Betriebe, Kinder und Erwachsene) verschiedene Untersuchungen im Bereich Stressregulation, Bewegung und Ernährung durchgeführt werden. Außerdem können Biofeedback-Trainings am Arbeitsplatz vorgenommen werden. Die wissenschaftlichen Grundlagen zu diesem Laborkonzept sind in Balzer und Stueck (2019) „Einführung in die Chrono-Bio-Psychologie" beschrieben und beruhen hauptsächlich auf der chronobiologischer Regulationsdiagnostik, die von Balzer und Hecht (1989, 2000) entwickelt wurden. Erste Erfahrungen mit dem Konzept der Mobilen Labordiagnostik wurden mit Expeditionen zu 8000er-Bergen im Himalaya (Cho Oyu, Gasherbrum 1 und 2 in 1996, 1998, 2002) und in die Anden (Aconcagua, Sangay-Expedition in 1995, 1996) bzw. durch Forschungen zum Kinderyoga (von 1993 bis 1997) und zu Biodanza (in 1998) gesammelt. Wir mussten für diese Unternehmungen eine mobile physiologische und psychoneuroimmunologische Labordiagnostik entwickeln, die leicht transportierbar und doch robust war und die mit einfachen psychologischen Skalen interpretierbar war (Balzer & Stueck, 2013; Balzer, Hecht, & Stueck, 1997; Kleessen, Schroedl, Stueck, Richter, Rieck & Krueger, 2005; Sack, 2012; Sack et al., 2004a, 2004b; Stueck & Schröder, 1995; Stueck, Balzer, Hecht, Schröder, & Rigotti, 2005; Stueck, Villegas, Perche, & Balzer, 2007; Stueck & Villegas, 2008; Villegas et al., 1999). Diese mobilen Laborforschungen in Extrembereichen wurden dann auf stark belastete Berufsfelder, z.B. im pädagogischen Bereich (Mueller, Stueck, & Balzer, 2014; Stueck, Hörnig, & Hecht, 2001; Stueck & Sonntag, 2005; Stueck, Rigotti, & Balzer, 2005; Stueck, Sonntag, & Schoppe, 2011) bzw. Arbeitslose Patienten (Dressler, Huhn, & Stueck, 1999) übertragen.

## 2 Beispiele für Tests im Mobilen Gesundheitslabor

Einen Überblick über alle Prozeduren sind im Artikel „Gesundheitswürfel" (Stueck, 2019) veröffentlicht. Nachfolgend werden folgende ausgewählte Messprozeduren erläutert:

- Herzratenvariabilität (HRV) und Rhythmische Sinusarrhythmie (RSA)
- Stressdiagnostischer Test, 24-h-Monitoring mittels smardwatch-System
- Hautsensibilitätsmessung, Blutdruckentspannungstest und Cortisol-Stresstest

### 2.1 Herzratenvariabilität und Rhythmische Sinusarrhythmie

Mit Hilfe der HRV Messung besteht die Möglichkeit mit wenig Zeitaufwand und ohne große technische Anforderungen Aussagen zum Zustand der physiologischen Anpassungsfähigkeit eines Menschen zu treffen. Eine ausgewogene Veränderung der Herzfrequenz mit sinusartigem Verlauf kennzeichnet hierbei ein gutes Zusammenspiel des Sympathikus und Parasympathikus. Sind beide Bestandteile zu gleichen Anteilen ausgeprägt, gelingt es dem Körper sich eigenständig zu regulieren und an verschiedenen Anforderungen anzupassen. Bei Ungleichgewicht ist der Körper von einer Unfähigkeit zur neurovegetativen Anpassung gekennzeichnet, was wiederum perspektivisch zu einem verringerten Wohlbefinden führt.

Die Software-Lösung im Gesundheitsmobil bietet sowohl die Erhebung der Kurzzeit-HRV sowie eines 24h Monitorings als Analyse an. Erst beide Messungen in Kombination sowie die psychologische Diagnostik im Gesundheitswürfel ermöglicht eine Aussage zum derzeitigen Stressregulationszustand einer Person. Neben der HRV-Messung bietet das Gesundheitslabor zusätzlich noch die Möglichkeit die eigene HRV mit Hilfe der respiratorischen Sinusarrhythmie (RSA) zu trainieren und zu veranschaulichen. Die RSA kennzeichnet die Verbindung zwischen

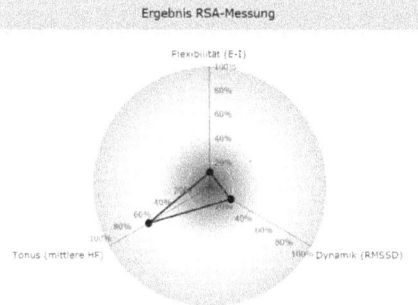
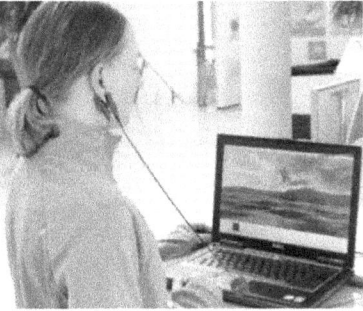

Abbildung 1. Ergebnisprotokoll der Rhythmischen Sinusarrythmiemessung und Biofeedback am Arbeitsplatz (Stress-Pilot, 2016).

Atmung und Herzfrequenz und ist dadurch gekennzeichnet, dass sich die Herzfrequenz erhöht, sobald man tief einatmet und die Herzfrequenz deutlich abfällt, wenn man ausatmet. Dieses Zusammenspiel aus Atmung und Veränderung der Herzfrequenz kann im mobilen Gesundheitslabor zu folgenden Diagnostik- und Übungszwecken verwendet werden:

a) Zunächst wird die RSA Leistung eines Probanden gemessen (Abb. 1), während sich an einer Atemhilfe orientiert. Dabei wird (1) der Parasympathische Grundtonus, (2) die Dynamik, d.h. die Schnelligkeit der Aktivierung des Parasympathikus (Stressbremse) und (3) die Flexibilität (Anpassungsfähigkeit des Herz-Kreislaufsystems) untersucht.

b) Im zweiten Schritt wird das Training des Probanden mittels Biofeedback-Messung angeboten (3 Minuten, Abbildung 1). In dieser Methode erhält der Proband über visuelle Marker den Hinweis wie gut die derzeitige Synchronisation von Atmung und Herzfrequenz ist. Das Biofeedbacksystem soll ermöglichen bislang unbewusste Körperfunktionen (Atmung, Herzschlag) zu veranschaulichen und bewusst zu steuern. Das Verhältnis von einem Atemzyklus (Ein- und Ausatmung) und 4 Herzschlägen ist optimal (Atempulsquotient).

Mit Hilfe dieser zweistufigen Analyse, Datenerhebung und Trainingseinheit werden den Probanden Möglichkeiten zur Verbesserung der eigenen Lebensqualität angeboten.

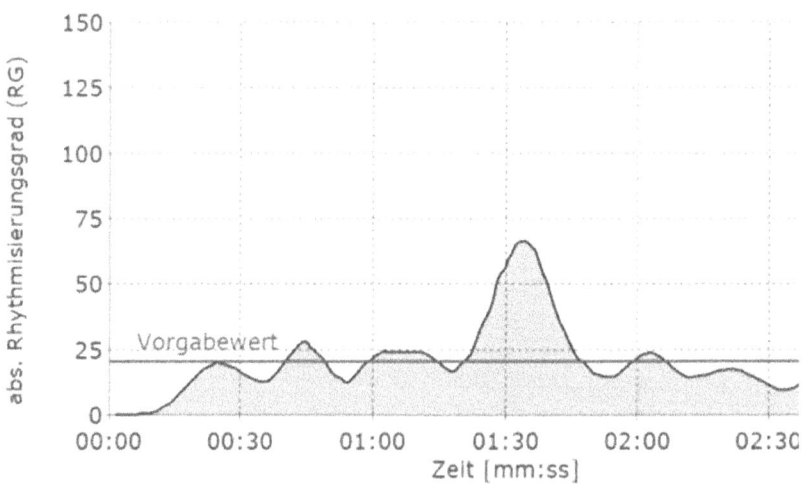

**Abbildung 2.** Ergebnis der Biofeedbackübung einer Probandin. Die Werte über der Linie (Vorgabewert) zeigen eine gelingende Synchronisierung an. Hier besteht Übungsbedarf.

## 2.2 Bestimmung der Veränderung der Perioden im chonobiologischen Stress-Entspannungs-Test (Chrono-bio-psychologische Regulationsdiagnostik)

Im Zusammenhang mit Untersuchungen zum Einfluss von Lärm-Stressoren auf den Menschen wurde von Balzer und Hecht (1989, 2000) der Stressentspannungstest (SET; Abb. 2) entwickelt. Der Stress-Entspannungstest wird mit der durch Balzer entwickelte smardwatch-System durchgeführt (s. Abb. 4). Diese Mess-Uhr (Abb. 3) kann folgende in Tabelle 1 dargestellte Parameter bestimmen.

Im SET soll sich der Proband 20 Minuten im „Liegenden Sitzen" entspannen. Nach 10 Minuten wird er durch einen akustischen Stressor (Lärm als „nichtkognitiver" Stressor) „gestört". Entscheidend für die Auswertung ist das Verhalten in der Stressor-Phase und danach. Über die Bestimmung von stabilen und instabilen

Tabelle 1. Mess-Parameter des smardwatch-Systems

| Messparameter | Zuordnung |
|---|---|
| 3D-Beschleunigung | Verhalten |
| 3D-Lage | Verhalten |
| Elektromyogramm | Muskelaktivität |
| Hautwiderstand | vegetativ-emotionale Reaktion |
| Hautpotential | vegetativ-nervale Reaktion |
| Hauttemperatur | metabolische Reaktion |

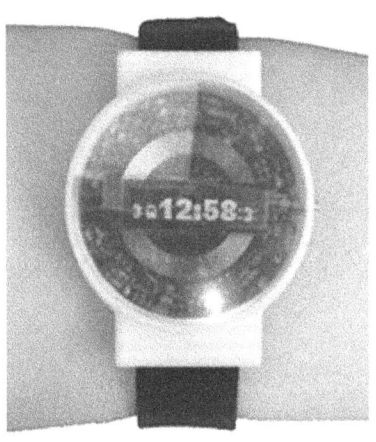

Abbildung 3. Smardwatch-System (rechts) als Uhr mit 24-h-Biofeedback-Monitoring.

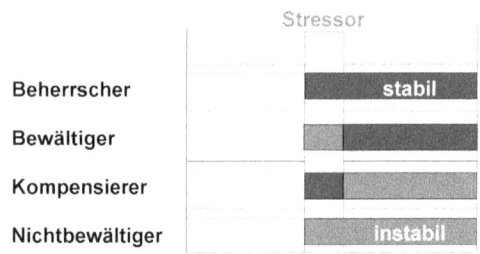

**Abbildung 4.** Klassifikation von vier Stresstypen im SET.

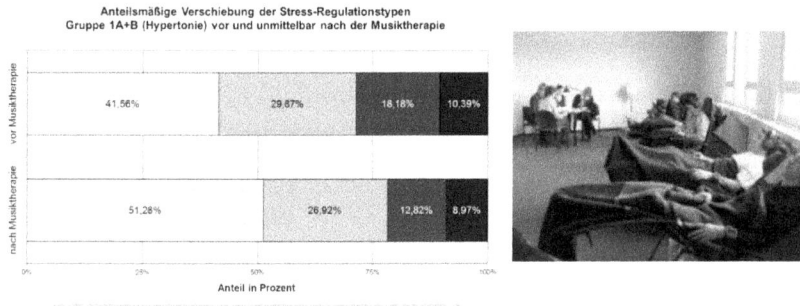

**Abbildung 5.** Stressregulationstypen von Klienten mit Hypertonie ($n$ = 32) vor und nach musiktherapeutischer Intervention (Balzer, 2006).
*Mittelwert über drei vegetativen Reaktionen (muskuläre, vegetativ-emotionale und vegetativ-nervale Reaktion).*

Phasen eines der vegetativen Parameter (Hautwiderstand/HW, Hautpotenzial/HP, Elektromyogramm/EMG) gestattet die Chrono-Biopsychologische Regulationsdiagnostik (CBR) einen Zugang zur Bestimmung von vier verschiedenen Reaktionsmustern bzgl. des Umgangs mit Stressoren (Abb. 4).

Mit diesem Testverfahren ist es auch möglich den Erfolg einer Behandlung oder von Betrieblichen Gesundheitsmaßnahmen nachzuweisen. Dazu wird der Test unter Beachtung chronobiologischer Regeln wiederholt angewendet. In der Regel vor Beginn und nach der Intervention (Abbildung 5).

## 2.3 Chronobiologisches 24-Stunden Monitoring

Mit dem smardwatch-System können in verschiedenen Situationen (während des Autofahrens, beim Musizieren zur Messung von Podiumsangst, Entspannungstherapie, s. Abbildung 6 von links nach rechts) die in Tabelle 1 genannten Parameter

Das mobile Gesundheitslabor 79

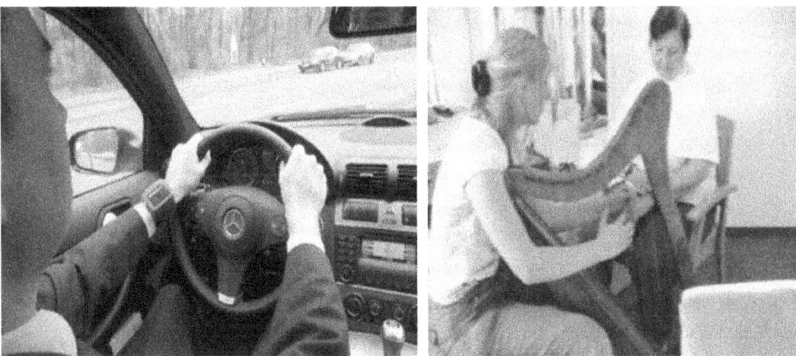

**Abbildung 6.** Stressmessungen mit smardwatch-System mit verschiedenen Zielgruppen

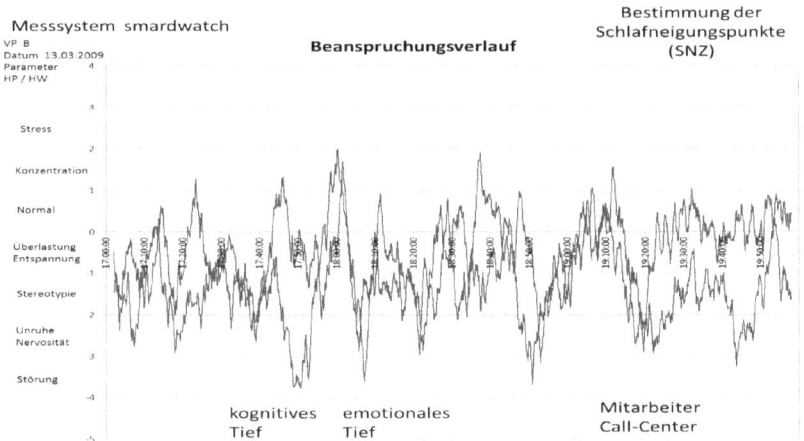

**Abbildung 7.** Auftreten von emotionalen und kognitiven Schlafneigungszeitpunkten.

in einer Laufzeit von 5 Tagen (ohne Akku-Nachladung) registriert werden. Eine interne Zwischenspeicherung der Messdaten von ca. 10h sowie eine telemetrische Datenübertragung via WLAN ermöglichen eine kontinuierliche Datenaufzeichnung. Für die Datenauswertung steht eine gerätespezifische Software (Chronomar, 2016) zur Verfügung.

Beispielhaft zeigen Langzeituntersuchungen bei einer Mitarbeiterin eines Call Centers (Abbildung 7), dass in Abhängigkeit von den Belastungen, die Zahl der Erschöpfungsmomente (Kognitive bzw. Emotionale Tiefs und Schlafneigungspunkte) zunehmen und sich der zeitliche Abstand zwischen ihnen verkürzt.

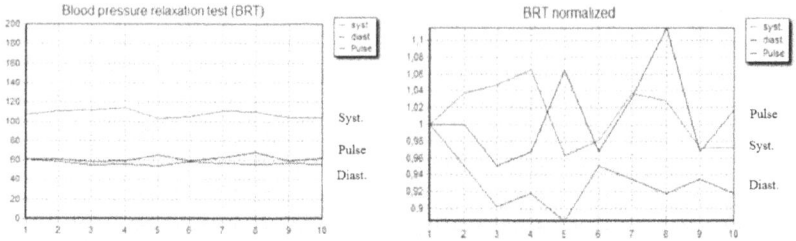

**Abbildung 8.** Veränderung des Blutdrucks während des Blutdruck-Entspannungstests (BET); links: Originalwerte [mmHg] im 10-min-Verlauf, rechts: normierte Werte.

## 2.4 Bestimmung der Blutdruckveränderung als chronobiologisches Prozess-Maß für Entspannungsfähigkeit – Blutdruck-Entspannungstest

Beim Blutdruck-Entspannungstest (BET) wird der Proband gebeten sich bequem zu setzen und sich mit hoch gelegten Füßen zu entspannen bzw. sich auf die eigene Atmung zu konzentrieren. Innerhalb der nächsten 10 Minuten (pro Minute jeweils eine Messung) wird der Blutdruck (systolisch, diastolisch) und Puls gemessen. Aus dem Verlauf der normierten systolischen Werte wird eine Entspannungskurve mittels Regression berechnet (Abbildung 8). Der Exponent der Näherungsfunktion wird als BET Grad ausgegeben. Je größer dieser Wert ist, desto höher ist die Entspannungsfähigkeit. Negative Werte bedeuten hierbei Erregung statt Entspannung. Anhand der Normwerte teilt eine Software die jeweilige Testperson in Normotoniker, Hypotoniker oder Hypertoniker ein. Die psychologische Beurteilung der systolischen Blutdruckwerte für die 3 Gruppen wurde in einem Forschungsprojekt mit Lehrern herausgearbeitet (Stueck, Sonntag, & Schoppe, 2011; Stueck, Rigotti, Roudini, Galindo, & Utami, 2016).

Eine weitere Möglichkeit der Auswertung dieser Daten bzgl. der Selbstentspannungsfähigkeit des Blutdrucks stellt die von Stueck und Lander im Psychologischen Institut der Universität Leipzig entwickelte Methode der empirischen Ausgleichsfunktion zur Beschreibung von Entspannungsverläufen im Blutdruck-Entspannungstest dar (Hecht, Andler, Breinl, Voigt-Spychala, Stueck, & Lander, 2001)[1].

---

1 Die exponentielle Ausgleichsfunktion hat allgemein die Form: y=a+b exp (ct) mit: a als Amplitude, b als maximales Gefälle, a+b als Achsenabschnitt [y(t=0)], c als Steilheit der Funktion. Diese Steilheit der Funktion (c) stellt den eigentlichen Veränderungsparameter dar und kann interpretiert werden.

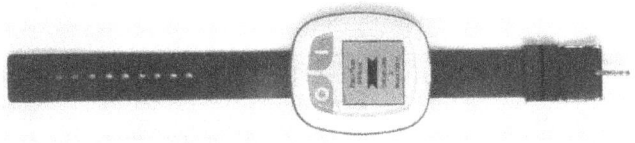

Abbildung 9. Testsystem *sensirec zur Bestimmung von unspezifischer Hypersensibilität*

## 2.5 Ableitung von Gesundheits- und Krankheitsprozessen mittels der Bestimmung der Hypersensibilität der Haut

In den eingangs erwähnten Untersuchungen zum Stresserleben in Extremsituationen von Himalaja- und Anden-Expeditionen in den 90er Jahren wurden Hypersensibilitätszustände entdeckt (Balzer & Stueck, 2013, 2019; Stueck, Balzer, Hecht, Schröder, & Rigotti, 2005). Diese regulationsdiagnostischen Begleitzustände bei der Messung der Elektrodermalen Aktivität bzw. des Hautwiderstandes spielen bei chronischen Stresszuständen bzw. bei Burnout-Zuständen eine wichtige Rolle. Es wurde daraufhin eine Mess-Prozedur (Sensirec) entwickelt, mit der die Zustände abbildbar sind (s. Abbildung 9).

Folgende Befunde zur, mit sensirec gemessenen, Hypersensibilität liegen bisher vor:

- häufigere Hypersensibilität bei Synästhetikern (Schneider, Stueck, & Hecht, 2001),
- Korrelationen zu frühkindlichen Traumata (Leitner, Stueck, & Balzer, 2015),
- Korrelationen zu dysfunktionalen Einstellungen (Mueller, Stueck, & Balzer, 2014),
- reduzierte Empathie bei hypersensiblen Lehrern (Stueck et al., 2004; Stueck & Villegas, 2008),
- 90% der direkt Erdbeben-Betroffenen (Hausverlust, Todesfall) in Nepal 2014 waren hypersensibel (Stueck, Utami, Boehm, & Balzer, 2016),
- Zusammenhang von Hyposensibilität und erfragten Hypersensibilitätsreaktionen: Licht, Lärm, Gerüche, Schmerz (Stueck, Balzer, & Utami, 2019),
- Zusammenhang von psychomotorischer Hyperaktivität (Schrittzahl) mit gemessener Hyper- bzw. Hyposensibilität (Stueck, Balzer, & Utami, 2019),
- Geringeres Raum-Wohlbefinden bei Hypersensibilität (Stueck, Balzer, & Utami, 2019),
- Absinken der Hypersensibilität bei erfolgreicher Gipfel-Besteigung (Stueck, 2015),
- Zusammenhang Hypersensiblität, Typ-S, Stressmustern (Stueck et al., 2001, 2005; Tab. 2).

Tabelle 2. Aktivierung und Hypersensibilität (Stueck et al., 2005)

| Typ | Aktivierung | Deaktivierung | verteilte Aktivierung | Hypersensibilität |
|---|---|---|---|---|
| Typ-S / Schonung | .38* | -.41* | -.34'* | .52** |
| Typ-A / Überforderung | -.27 | .20 | .29 | -.36 |
| Typ-G / Gesundheit | -.10 | -.05 | .16 | -.10 |
| Typ B / Burnout | .12 | .02 | -.17 | .14 |

* p<.10, ** p<.05 (einseitig), N = 20 / Typen = AVEM nach Schaarschmidt (2006)

**Wie kann Hypersensibilität abgebaut werden?**
Es konnte nachgewiesen werden, das Hypersensibilität durch Biodanza (Versuchsgruppe in Argentinien und Deutschland) und durch Meditation (Synästhesie) (Stueck & Villegas, 2008; Stueck, Villegas, Perche, & Balzer, 2007) abgebaut werden konnte. In einer Studie in Lettland (Raikova, 2016) war die Drop Out Rate erhöht bei Personen mit Hypersensibilität. Hypersensible Versuchspersonen, die zum Typ Schonung gehören, verblieben dagegen in einer Versuchsgruppe.

Zusammenfassend können folgende Erklärungsmodelle für Hypersensibilität angenommen werden (Balzer & Stueck, 2019):

a) *Stufenmodell der Erschöpfung des Organismus unter Belastungsdruck* (s. Abb. 10): Dieses Modell zeigt, dass die Normosensitivität mit einer gelingenden Autoregulation zusammenhängt. Bei steigendem Belastungsdruck kommt es zur Hypersensibilität und bei weiter anhaltender Belastung zu einem Sprung in hyposensible Zustände. Es stellte sich heraus, dass die hyposensiblen Zustände mit Erschöpfungszuständen zusammenhängen.

b) *Vulnerabilitätsmodell der Hypersensibilität* (s. Abb. 11): Der Effekt-Mechanismus dieses Vulnerabilitätsmodells könnte auf dem Zusammenhang zwischen der Leistungsfähigkeit, der Leistungserbringung, dem Grad der Sensibilität und dem Erregungs- bzw. Entspannungszustand einer Person basieren. Zu Beginn einer Entspannung – ausgehend vom Punkt 0 in Abbildung 10 – kann die Sensibilität ansteigen, ohne gewöhnlich jedoch den Bereich der Hypersensibilität (rot, s. Abb. 11) zu erreichen (grün). Der rote Bereich wird nur beim Vorliegen von Stress erreicht. Nach dem Auslösen einer tiefen Entspannung, dem „Abschalten", können Zustände der Hyposensibilität auftreten (blau). Darüber hinaus kann die Hyposensibilität auch infolge Überbeanspruchung durch Erschöpfung oder Burnout entstehen (s. Abb. 11).

Hypersensibilität bzw. Hyposensibilität kann ebenso Veranlagung sein. Es wird angenommen, dass Menschen, die hochsensibel veranlagt oder entwickelt sind (z.B. Künstler), unter Stressoren-Einfluss schneller in den Bereich der Hypersensibilität und nachfolgend – in Folge Erschöpfung - in den Bereich der Hyposensibilität

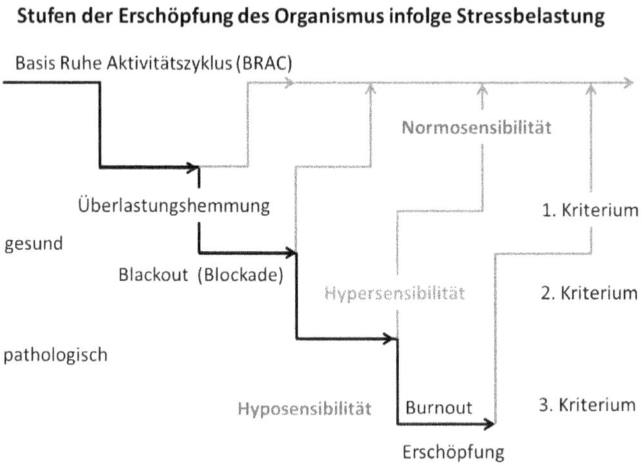

Das mobile Gesundheitslabor 83

**Stufen der Erschöpfung des Organismus infolge Stressbelastung**

Basis Ruhe Aktivitätszyklus (BRAC)

Normosensibilität

gesund — Überlastungshemmung — 1. Kriterium

Blackout (Blockade) — Hypersensibilität — 2. Kriterium

pathologisch

Hyposensibilität | Burnout — 3. Kriterium

Erschöpfung

**Abbildung 10.** Einordnung der Hyper – und Hyposensibilität in das Stufen-Modell der Erschöpfung des Organismus (Balzer & Stueck, 2013; Stueck et al., 2005).

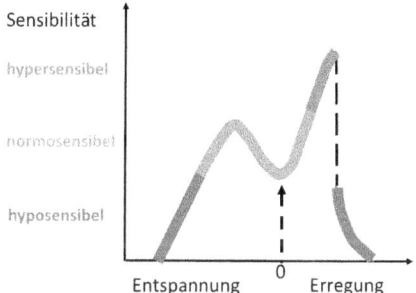

**Abbildung 11.** Zusammenhang zwischen Sensibilität, Entspannung und Erregung.

geraten. Aufgrund der Stress- und Erschöpfungszustände kann Hypo- und Hypersensibilität als vulnerabler Zustand bezeichnet werden, der die Anfälligkeit, bestimmte Krankheiten auszuprägen, erhöht. Das Gegenteil von Vulnerabilität ist die Resilienz (Widerstandsfähigkeit), sie liegt bei Normosensibilität vor. Personen, die als vulnerabel gelten, d.h. die hypo- und hypersensibel getestet werden, sind emotional leichter anfällig und können leichter psychische Störungen entwickeln (Wenninger & Boos, 2003). Es wird nach unseren Studien außerdem angenommen, dass der Übergang von hypersensibel, d.h. von sehr starker Erregung, zu hyposensibel sprunghaft erfolgt (s. Abb.11).

Interpretation der Sensirec-Messungen ist nur mit psychologischen Skalen möglich. Die Hypersensibilitätsmessungen sollten mit erfragten Hypersensibilitätszuständen (Skala zur Hypersensibilität; Stueck, Balzer, & Utami, 2019) oder anderen psychologischen Skalen des Gesundheitswürfels (Stueck, 2019) interpretiert werden. So fanden Stueck, Balzer, & Utami (2019), dass das unangenehme Erleben von Arbeitslärm, von Schmerz, von Lichtempfindung mit Hyposensibilität korreliert. Die Gründe dafür könnte sein, dass hyposensible Personen aufgrund ihrer Erschöpfung gar keine Sensibilität mehr aufbauen können. Mit dem 24-Stunden-Monitorings mit dem smardwatch-System (s.2.3) können diese Ermüdungspunkte nachgewiesen werden.

## 2.6 Ableitung stressrelevanter Prozesse mittels der Bestimmung von Cortisol

Cortisol ist ein Stresshormon an dessen Tagesrhythmik (schrittweise Reduktion zu vier Messzeitpunkten 8,9,15,18 Uhr) erkennbar wird, wie die Stressverarbeitung einer Person erfolgt. Eine gestörte Rhytmik ist z.b. bei Depressionen nachweisbar (Gatti, Antonelli, Prearo, Spinella, Cappellin, & De Palo, 2009; Nicolson, 2008). Diese circadiane psychoneurimmunologische Stressdiagnostik ist ebenso Bestandteil des mobilen Gesundheitslabors, sowie eine einfache Ernährungs- und Bewegungsdiagnostik.

# 3 Zusammenfassende Bemerkungen

In diesem Artikel wird ein Laborkonzept beschrieben, welches transportabel und relativ preiswert ist und spezifische Aussagen zu autonomen Verarbeitungsweisen des Individuums unter Belastungsdruck treffen kann. Die psychobiologischen Beanspruchungszustände werden im Mobilen Gesundheitslabor mit zwei Hauptmodulen bestimmt:

a) verschiedenen leicht aufbauaren Messprozeduren als Einpunkt-Messung und
b) längere prozesshafte Untersuchungen der Beanspruchungsmuster über die Zeit.

Diese psychobiologischen Zustandsbestimmungen werden im mobilen Gesundheitslabor immer mit Hilfe der psychologischen Diagnostik der Gesundheitswürfeldiagnostik (s. Stueck, 2019) interpretiert. Insofern sollte das mobile Gesundheitslabor als Teil des Gesundheitswürfelkonzeptes angesehen werden, welches mit sehr vielen belasteten Berufsgruppen angewendet werden kann.

# 4 Affiliations

Prof. Dr. Marcus Stueck
Institution: DPFA-Akademie für Arbeitsgesundheit/International Research Academy – BIONET
Address: DPFA-Weiterbildung GmbH, Täubchenweg 83, 04317 Leipzig, Germany.
E-mail: marcus.stueck@dpfa-hs.de

Dr. Hans-Ullrich Balzer
Institution: Institut Agrar-u. Stadtökologische Projekte an der Humboldt-Universität Berlin
Address: Lebenswissenschaftliche Fakultät, Humboldt-Universität zu Berlin, Philippstraße 13, Haus 16, 10115 Berlin, Germany.
E-mail: ullrich.balzer@agrar.hu-berlin.de

B. A. Sebastian Mueller
Institution: International Research Academy - BIONET
Address: Leipziger Str. 64, 04420 Markranstädt, Germany.
E-mail: sebastian.mueller@bildungsgesundheit.de

Dr. Dian Sari Utami
Institution: Department of Psychology, Islamic University of Indonesia
Address: Jalan Kaliurang km 14.5, Sleman, 55584 Daerah Istimewa Yogyakarta, Indonesia.
E-mail: dian.utami@uii.ac.id

Prof. Dr. Ulrich Sack
Institution: Institut für Klinische Immunologie, Medizinische Fakultät, Universität Leipzig.
Address: Johannisallee 30, Haus J, 04103 Leipzig, Germany.
E-mail: sack@uni-leipzig.de

# 5 Referenzliste

Balzer, H.-U. (2002). *Auswertungen von 24 h-Stundenmessungen der vegetativen Regulation von Paaren.* Unpublished manuscript, Humboldt Universität zu Berlin, Berlin.

Balzer, H.-U. (2006). *System Smardwatch.* Unpublished manuscript, Humboldt Universität zu Berlin, Berlin.

Balzer, H.-U. (2009). Chronobiology – as a foundation for and an approach to a new understanding of the influence of music. In R. Haas & V. Brandes (Eds.), *Music that works: Contributions of biology, neurophysiology, psychology, sociology, medicine and musicology* (pp. 25–81). Wien, New York: Springer.

Balzer, H.-U., & Hecht, K. (1989). Ist Stress noninvasiv zu messen? Wissenschaftliche Zeitschrift der Humboldt-Universität Berlin. *Reihe Medizin,* 38(4), 456–460.

Balzer, H.-U., & Hecht, K. (2000). Chrono-Psychobiologische Regulationsdiagnostik (CRD) – Ein neuer Weg zur objektiven Bestimmung von Gesundheit und Krankheit. In K. Hecht & H.-U. Balzer, *Stressmanagement, Katastrophenmedizin, Regulationsmedizin, Prävention* (S. 134–154). Lengerich: Pabst Science Publishers.

Balzer, H.-U., & Stueck, M. (2013). The psychobiological meaning and measuring of hypersensibility. *Biopsychological Basics of Life, 2,* 46–52.

Balzer, H.-U., & Stueck, M. (2019). *Einführung in Chronobiopsychologie.* Manuscript submitted for publication.

Balzer, H.-U., Hecht, K, & Stueck, M. (1997, February). *Stress diagnostic control of efficiency during Yoga Training on stressed school children.* Paper session presented at the 9th International Montreux Congress on Stress, Montreux.

Chronomar. (2016). *Chronobiologisches Monitoring – Analyse und Regulation.* Retrieved on December 15, 2018 from http://www.chronomar.de/index.html

Dressler, T., Huhn, B., & Stueck, M. (1999). Untersuchungen zum Stresserleben von Patienten mit dem Stress-Entspannungstest (SET). In S. Dauer & H. Hennig (Hrsg.), *Arbeitslosigkeit und Gesundheit* (S. 176–193). Halle (Saale): Mitteldeutscher Verlag.

Gatti, R., Antonelli, G., Prearo, M., Spinella, P., Cappellin, E., & De Palo, E. F. (2009). Diagnostic laboratory procedures (Cortisol) in human biological fluids. *Clinical Biochemistry, 42,* 1205–1217.

Hecht, K., Andler, S., Breinl, S., Voigt-Spychala, C., Stueck, M., & Lander, H.-J. (2001). Objektive Kontrolle der Selbstentspannungsfähigkeit mittels Zeitreihenmessungen des Blutdrucks und der Elektrodermalen Aktivität (EDA). In K. Hecht, H.-P. Scherf & O. König (Hrsg.), *Emotioneller Stress durch Überforderung und Unterforderung* (S. 253–272). Strasburg: Schibri-Verlag.

Kleessen, B., Schroedl, W., Stueck, M., Richter, A., Rieck, O., & Krueger, M. (2005). Mokrobial and immunological responses relative to high altitude exposure in mountaineers. *Journal of Medicine & Science in Sports & Exercise, 37*(8), 1313–1318.

Leitner, S., Stueck, M., & Balzer, H.-U. (2015). *Hypersensibilität und Erzieherinnengesundheit.* Unpublished manuscript, International Reseach Academy – Bionet, Leipzig.

Mueller, S., Stueck, M., & Balzer, H.-U. (2014). Zusammenhang von Biografie, Stress & Körperreaktionen bei Erziehern: Psycho-physiologische Laboruntersuchungen zur Erziehergesundheit. *ErgoMed Practische Arbeitsmedizin, 6,* 24–30.

Nicolson, N. A. (2008). Measurement of cortisol. In L. J. Luecken & L. C. Gallo (Eds.), *Handbook of Physiological Research Methods in Health Psychology* (pp. 37–74). Thousand Oaks, CA: Sage Publications, Inc.

Raikova, A. (2016). *Biodanza, Hypersensibility and Stress* (Unpublished master thesis). Riga Teacher Management Academy, Latvia.

Sack, U. (2012, October). *Psychoneuroimmunology and stress.* Paper session presented at the 1st Bionet International Conference, Riga. Retrieved on July 22, 2018 from http://www.bionet.name

Sack, U., Meier, K., Bauer, K., & Stueck, M. (2004a, December). *Psychoimmunological evaluation of stress prevention by Biodanza.* Paper session presented at the 3rd Leipzig Research Festival for Life Sciences, Zwickau.

Sack, U., Meier, K., Bauer, K., & Stueck, M. (2004b, September). *Psychoimmunological evaluation of stress preventive intervention programmes*. Poster session presented at the 7th Congress of the International Society of Neuro-Immunology, Venice.

Schaarschmidt, U. (2006). AVEM - ein persönlichkeitsdiagnostisches Instrument für die berufsbezogene Rehabilitation. In Arbeitskreis Klinische Psychologie in der Rehabilitation BDP (Hrsg.), *Psychologische Diagnostik - Weichenstellung für den Reha-Verlauf* (S. 59–82). Bonn: Deutscher Psychologen Verlag GmbH.

Schneider, S., Stueck, M., & Hecht, K. (2001). Synästhesiediagnose unter psychobiologischem Aspekt: Hypersensibilitätszustände der Elektrodermalen Aktivität (Pilotstudie). In K. Hecht, H.-P. Scherf & O. König (Hrsg.), *Emotioneller Stress durch Überforderung und Unterforderung* (S. 273–284). Strasburg: Schibri-Verlag.

Stress-Pilot. (2016, Juni). *Firma Biocomfort Diagnostics – HRV-Biofeedback*. Retrieved on July 22, 2018 from http://www.herzratenvariabilitaet.de/HRV-Geraete/Stress-Pilot.htm

Stueck, M. (2002, November). *Das meditative Bergsteigen einer chilenischen Mt. Everest-Expedition (8848 Meter): Eine Pilotstudie zum Einsatz von Entspannungsmethoden und Meditation beim Höhenbergsteigen*. Paper session presented at Kongressband Symposium Psyche und Berg, Schneeberg.

Stueck, M. (2015). *Wissenschaftliche Studie zur Zweitbesteigung des Pik Leipzig in Kirgistan/Pamir (5725 m)*. Unpublished Manuscript, International Research Academy-Bionet, Leipzig.

Stueck, M. (2019). Der Gesundheitswürfel. In E. Witruk & D. S. Utami, *Studies of Educational and Rehabilitation Psychology, vol. 8: Traumatic experiences and dyslexia*. Manuscript submitted for publication.

Stueck, M., & Sonntag, A. (2005). Normativ auffälliges Beanspruchungserleben von Lehrern. *ErgoMed Practische Arbeitsmedizin, (4),* 105–113.

Stueck, M., & Villegas, A. (2008). Zur Gesundheit tanzen? Empirische Forschungen zu Biodanza. Strasburg: Schibri-Verlag.

Stueck, M., Balzer, H.-U., & Mueller, S. (2014). Zusammenhang von Biografie, Stress & Körperreaktion bei Erziehern: Psycho-physiologische Laboruntersuchungen zur Erziehergesundheit. *ErgoMed Praktische Arbeitsmedizin, 6(38),* 24–30.

Stueck, M., Balzer, H.-U., & Utami, D. S. (2019). *Studies and psychological interpretations about measured hypersensibility*. Manuscript submitted for publication.

Stueck, M., Balzer, H.-U., Hecht, K., & Schröder, H. (2004, August). *Psychophysiological investigation of a high mountain expedition to Cho-Oyu (Tibet, 8201 m)*. Paper session presented at the 28th International Congress of Psychology, Beijing.

Stueck, M., Balzer, H.-U., Hecht, K., Schröder, H., & Rigotti T. (2005). Psychological and Psychophysiological effects of a High-Mountains Expedition to Tibet. *Journal of Human Performance in Extreme Environments*, 8(1–2), 11–20.

Stueck, M., Hecht, K., Schröder, H., & Rieck, O. (2001). Emotionell – vegetative Regulation unter Höhenhypoxie und extremen Lebensbedingungen des Hochgebirges (Cho Oyu 8205m). In K. Hecht, H.-P. Scherf & O. Koenig (Hrsg.), *Emotioneller Stress durch Überforderung und Unterforderung* (S. 421–442). Strasburg: Schibri-Verlag.

Stueck, M., Hörnig, D., & Hecht, K. (2001). Lehrerbelastung unter dem Aspekt psychologischer und chronobiologischer Regulationsdiagnostik. In K. Hecht, H. -P. Scherf & O. König (Hrsg.), *Emotioneller Stress durch Überforderung und Unterforderung* (S. 383–402). Strasburg: Schibri-Verlag.

Stueck, M., Meyer, K., Bauer, K., & Sack, U. (2002, September). *Psychoimmunological process Evaluation of a stress preventive intervention program for teachers*. Poster session presented at 33. Jahrestagung der Gesellschaft für Immunologie, Marburg.

Stueck, M., Rigotti, T., & Balzer, H.-U. (2005). Wie reagieren Lehrer bei Belastungen? Berufliche Bewältigungsmuster und psychophysiologische Korrelate. *Psychologie in Erziehung und Unterricht, 52*, 250–260.

Stueck, M., Rigotti, T., Roudini, J., Galindo, E., & Utami, D. S. (2016). Relationship between blood pressure and psychic features of experience and behaviour among teachers. *Health Psychology Report, 4*(2), 128–136.

Stueck, M., Sonntag, A., & Schoppe, S. (2011). Systolischer Blutdruck und gesundheitspsychologische Eigenschaften bei Lehrern. *ErgoMed Practische Arbeitsmedizin, 2*, 44–52.

Stueck, M., und Schröder, H. (1995). *Erfolgsdruck lastete auf der Aconcagua Expedition*. Wissenschaftsteil der Leipziger Volkszeitung (S. 12), Leipzig.

Stueck, M., Utami, D. S., Boehm, M., & Balzer, H.-U. (2016, July). *Empirical study of psychological factors and intervention to increase psychological harmony after the earthquake in Nepal*. Paper session presented at the 31st International Congress of Psychology (ICP), organized by American Psychological Association (APA), Yokohama, Japan. Retrieved on August 23, 2018 from http://www.bionet.name

Stueck, M., Villegas, A., Bauer, K., Terren, R., Toro, V., & Sack, U. (2009). Psycho-Immunological Process Evaluation of Biodanza. *Signum Temporis Pedagogy & Psychology, 2*(1), 99–113. DOI: https://doi.org/10.2478/v10195-011-0024-7

Stueck, M., Villegas, A., Perche, F., & Balzer, H.-U. (2007). Neue Wege zum Stressabbau im Lehrerberuf: Biodanza und Yoga als körperorientierte Verfahren zur Reduktion psycho-vegetativer Spannungszustände. *ErgoMed Practische Arbeitsmedizin, 03*, 68–75.

Stueck, M., Villegas, A., Schröder, H., Sack, U., Bauer, K., Terren, R., ... & Toro, R. (2004, September). *Psycho-neuro-immunologische Effekte einer neuen bewegungs- und körperorientierten Interventionsmethode zur Förderung des Identitätsausdrucks und der Autoregulation (Biodanza)*. Poster session presented at 44. Kongress der Deutschen Gesellschaft für Psychologie, Goettingen.

Villegas, A., Stueck, M., Terren, R., Toro, V., Schröder, H., Balzer, H.-U., ... Mazzarella, L. (1999). Psychologische und Physiologische Wirkungen von Biodanza. *Revista Conexión Abierta, 2*, 15–18.

Wenninger, K., & Boos, A. (2003). Behandlung erwachsener Opfer sexuellen Kindesmissbrauchs. In A. Maerker (Hrsg.), *Therapie der Postraumatischen Belastungsstörung* (S. 176–184). Berlin, Heidelberg: Springer.

Marcus Stueck

# Der Gesundheitswürfel: Ein Instrument zur Psychischen Gefährdungs- und Ressourcenbeurteilung im Rahmen des Biozentrischen und Betrieblichen Gesundheitsmanagements in Unternehmen und Institutionen

**Abstract:** The Health Cube is a scientifically evaluated instrument of reflection and evidence-based intervention in the context of the Biocentric Occupational Health management and Workplace Health Promotion. It can be used to detect factors that hinder employee health in companies and institutions, as well as of other target groups (e.g. teachers, professional drivers and use in crisis areas). There are different versions for use: in group discussions, as questionnaires, as a biofeedback cube for the self-control of physiological stress states. There are six levels of cubes to make evidence-based analyzes with a traffic light system for people and institutions to necessary behavioral and health interventions: (1) work factors, (2) psychobiological states, (3) stress-psychological reactions, (4) internal and external resources, (5) biocentric health parameters, and (6) behavioral and environmental prevention and health promotion. In the process, an individual's intrinsic motivation towards health and life (so called Biocentric Health Commitment, Self-care) is developed in order to remain healthy without simply imitating the company's health goals. The mobile health diagnostic laboratory (level 2) in the health cube is based on the development of chrono-bio-psychological as well as on nutritional and movement diagnostic and psycho-neuro-immunological procedures. The concept is constantly being scientifically evaluated and developed and used nationally and internationally.

**Keywords:** risk assessment of mental stress, biocentric occupational health management, evidence-based workplace biocentric health promotion, complex research tool of work and organizational psychology

**Zusammenfassung:** Der Gesundheitswürfel ist ein wissenschaftlich evaluiertes Instrument der Reflexion und evidenzbasierten Intervention im Rahmen des biozentrischen betrieblichen Gesundheitsmanagements und der betrieblichen Gesundheitsförderung. Es kann verwendet werden, um Faktoren zu ermitteln, die die Gesundheit von Mitarbeitern in Unternehmen und Institutionen sowie von anderen Zielgruppen (z. B. Lehrer, Berufskraftfahrer) einschränken. Es gibt verschiedene Versionen für den Einsatz: als workshop, Fragebogen, Biofeedback-Würfel zur Selbstkontrolle physiologischer Stresszustände. Es gibt sechs Würfel-Ebenen, um evidenzbasierte Analysen mit einem Ampelsystem für Personen und

Institutionen durchzuführen: (1) Arbeitsfaktoren, (2) psychobiologische Zustände, (3) stresspsychologische Reaktionen, (4) interne und externe Ressourcen, (5) biozentrisches Gesundheitsmanagement und (6) Verhaltens- und Verhältnisprävention. Dabei wird die intrinsische Motivation des Einzelnen in Bezug auf Gesundheit und Leben (biozentrische Selbstfürsorge) entwickelt, um gesund zu bleiben. Das mobile Gesundheitslabor (2) im Gesundheitswürfel basiert auf der Entwicklung chrono-bio-psychologischer sowie ernährungs- und bewegungsdiagnostischer und psycho-neuroimmunologischer Verfahren. Das Konzept wird ständig wissenschaftlich evaluiert (national und international) und weiterentwickelt.

**Schlüsselwörter:** Gefährdungsbeurteilung psychischer Belastungen, Biozentrisches betriebliches Gesundheitsmanagement, Evidenzbasierte betriebliche biozentrische Gesundheitsförderung, komplexes Untersuchungsinstrument der Arbeits- und Organisationspsychologie

# 1 Gefährdungsbeurteilung psychischer Belastungen und Gesundheitswürfel

Das Betriebliche Gesundheitsmanagement (BGM) und die Betriebliche Gesundheits-förderung (BGF) sind Prozeduren der Gestaltung, Lenkung und Entwicklung von Strukturen und Prozessen, um Arbeit bzw. die Organisation und das Verhalten am Arbeitsplatz gesundheitsförderlich zu gestalten, in folgenden Bereichen:

a) Stressregulation (Psychoedukation und Training zu stressrelevanten Themen)
b) Bewegungsförderung (u.a. Rückengerechtes Arbeiten, Bewegung in den Pausen)
c) Ernährung (Handlungswissen zu gesunder und zum Typ passender Ernährung)
d) Suchtprävention (Reflexion zu Sucht und Bewältigung, u.a. Alkohol, Medikamente).

Die Maßnahmen in diesen Bereichen, sollten nach einer Gefährdungsbeurteilung psychischer Belastungen (GPB) diagnosegeleitet geplant werden.
**Warum sollte die Gefährdungsbeurteilung (GPB) durchgeführt werden?** Durch die Gefährdungsbeurteilung sollen Behinderungen im Arbeitsalltag identifiziert werden, welche sich negativ auf die psychische Gesundheit auswirken können. Die Diagnosen psychischer Erkrankungen, aufgrund von Arbeits-Belastungen, haben in den letzten Jahren beständig zugenommen. Für Arbeitgeber bedeutet das v.a. lange Arbeitsunfähigkeitsphasen (Absentismus) oder das Arbeiten trotz Erkrankungen (Präsentismus), mit dem Auftreten chronischer Krankheiten. Deswegen ist es folgerichtig, dass das Arbeitsschutzgesetz seit 2014 alle deutschen Unternehmen explizit dazu verpflichtet, auch die psychischen Belastungen ihrer Beschäftigten bei der Arbeit zu ermitteln und zu dokumentieren, sowie entsprechende Arbeitsschutzmaßnahmen zu ergreifen[1].

---

1   u.a.: im Arbeitsschutzgesetz § 5, der Betriebssicherheitsverordnung § 3, Arbeitsstättenverordnung § 3.

**Was ist neu am Gesundheitswürfel?** Bisherige Instrumente zur Gefährdungsbeurteilung psychischer Belastungen (PGB) orientieren sich v.a. an der Analyse „krankmachender, äußerer" Arbeitsbedingungen und Risikofaktoren (Belastungen). Die Fragen sind zumeist willkürlich, ohne wissenschaftliche Validierung zusammengestellt. Auch innere Verarbeitungs-Vorgänge der Belastungen bzw. externale und internale Ressourcen werden bisher überhaupt nicht miterfasst oder aufgrund von Analysen interventiv entwickelt. Dadurch wird eine tiefere Reflexion nicht möglich und eine Möglichkeit der Entwicklung eines intrinsisch motivierten Gesundheitsverhaltens verschenkt. Es gibt Instrumente, die mit Zielerreichungsskalen überfrachtet sind, was wiederum eine Überforderung und kognitive Fokussierung auf das Problem darstellt und in der Praxis nachweislich nicht funktioniert, da beobachtbar ist, dass dadurch wenig effektiv eine Verhaltensänderung eintritt. Mit dem Gesundheitswürfel steht nun ein wissenschaftlich fundiertes, multidimensionales und multimethodales[2] Reflexionswerkzeug zur Verfügung (6 Ebenen, Abb. 4), welches auf Wunsch des Auftraggebers modulhaft, je nach Fragestellung zusammengesetzt werden kann und auch individuelle Verarbeitungs-besonderheiten in der Gefährdungsbeurteilung mitberücksichtigt, die in Beratungsge-sprächen verbalisiert werden können. Dadurch und durch die Tatsache, dass in 7 Inter-ventionsbereichen Maßnahmen abgeleitet werden können, ist der Beziehungs- und Inhaltsaspekt des Individuums zur Anforderung hin und bzgl. der Intervention balanciert (s. Fußnote 14). Mit einem normbasierten Ampelsystem (s. Abb. 4) können individualisiert oder gruppenspezifisch und punktgenau Präventions- und Gesundheitsförderungs-maßnahmen abgeleitet werden, wodurch das kostenintensive Gießkannenprinzip bei der Planung von Präventionsmaßnahmen vermieden wird (Stueck, Neumann, Mayer, Rillich, Dobrig, Lahm, Supplies, & Wallenhauer, 2010). Durch die Gesundheitswürfelmethode können in workshops oder als Fragebogen-Methode mit individualisierter oder gruppenspezifischer Auswertung Zusammenhänge zwischen Belastung und Beanspruchung erkannt und durch den Arbeitnehmer eine neue biozentrische Ebene im BGM entwickelt werden: Selbstfürsorge, Selbst-Empathie bzw. eigenverantwortliches Gesundheits-Engagement[3]. Diese Verhaltens-Ebene wird durch Skalen (u.a. Stueck, Schoppe, Lahn, & Toro, 2013) und durch das Erlebnis der Beeinflussbarkeit von Körperreaktionen im mobilen Gesundheitslabor angeregt (Ebene 2). Der Gesundheitswürfel ist so "ein Weg vom Innen nach Aussen": d.h. von der Selbstreflexion und Selbst-Empathie zu einem veränderten Umgang mit Belastungen. Die

---

[2] mehrere Methoden werden in ein Verfahren impliziert, Sachverhalt erhält unterschiedliche Perspektiven.
[3] Commitment to Health (CTH) geht auf das Modell der Verhaltensänderung von Prochaska und DiClemente (1982) zurück. Gesundheit wird dabei als optimales Wohlbefinden definiert. Biozentrische Betriebliche Gesundheitsförderung wurde von Stueck (2010) definiert und geht auf Arbeiten von Toro (2002) zurück.

Interventionseffekte von BGM-Maßnahmen können ebenfalls mit dem Gesundheitswürfel geprüft werden (Pre-Post-Analysen). Den Gesundheitswürfel gibt es als Fragebogen, Workshop-Variante und auch für Kinder-und Jugendliche (Stueck, 1997, 2011a).

## 2 Die Ebenen des Gesundheitswürfels

Zur Gefährdungbeurteilung psychischer Belastungen finden auf mehreren wählbaren Ebenen Messungen mit unterschiedlichen Methoden[4] statt.

### 2.1 Ebene 1: Analyse von Belastungen

Das ist die herkömmliche Gefährdungsanalyse, wobei die Psychischen Belastungen, d.h. alle Einflüsse, die von außen auf den Menschen psychisch einwirken[5], erfasst werden:

a. Allgemeine Belastungsanalyse, d.h. Identifizierung von Belastungen im Ist-Soll-Zustand im Arbeitsalltag (Abb. 1) (Molnar, Geißler-Gruber, & Haiden, 2011).
b) Spezielle Belastungsanalyse, z.B. für Berufskraftfahrer (Stueck et al., 2019), Pädagogen und Sozialarbeiter (Rudow, 2001; Stueck & Thinschmidt, 2010)[6].

### 2.2 Ebene 2: Bestimmung von psychobiologischen Beanspruchungszuständen und mustern (Mobiles Gesundheitslabor)

Arbeitsbelastungen (Ebene 1) lösen psychobiologische Beanspruchungszustände aus, die im mobil einsetzbaren Gesundheitslabor gemessen werden können (Balzer & Stueck, 2019)[7]:

---

4 Workshop (qualitative), Fragebogen (quantitative) mit ratingSkalen, standartisierten normierten Skalen, Projektive Testverfahren „Unternehmen als Fahrrad", „Unternehmen als Tier-Familie" und Farbdiagnostik, Polaritäten-Profil (Semantisches Differenzial). Zusätzlich einsetzbar. Repertory Grid Technik, um verdeckte Gesundheits-Einstellungen zu ermitteln und das mobile Gesundheitslabor (u.a. Stressdiagnostischer Test, s.1.2)
5 Rahmenbedingungen zu psychischen Belastungen beschreiben die Leitlinien der Deutschen Arbeitsschutz-strategie (GDA), des Arbeitsschutzgesetzes (§3, §5) und die Bundesanstalt für Arbeitsschutz und Arbeitsmedizin (BAuA) bzw. der Normenausschuss Ergonomie im Deutschen Institut für Normung e.V.
6 Bereiche: Kinder/Gruppen, Leitung/Arbeitsklima, Mittel, Arbeitsbedingungen, Körperliche Anforderungen.
7 Die Befunde und Messungen sind nur mit Hilfe der psychologischen Diagnostik (Ausdauer/Konzentration auf Arbeitsaufgaben) bzw. mit den Erhebungen der EBENE 3 (Beanspruchungsfolgen) interpretierbar.

Der Gesundheitswürfel 95

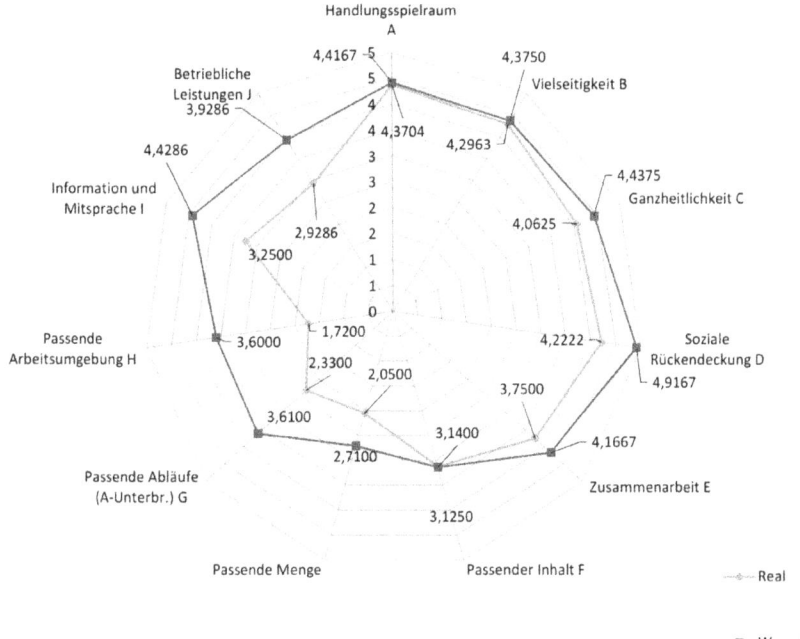

**Abbildung 1.** Beispiel einer Allgemeinen Arbeitsanalyse im GH-Würfel Ebene 1. *zusätzlich werden erfragt: Personalbesetzung, Arbeitszufriedenheit und Arbeitsklima, Work-Life-Balance.*

a) Physische und psychische Beanspruchungs-Zustände (als Einpunkt-Messung):
   a) Stressregulation: Blutdruck-Entspannungstest (Entspannungsfähigkeit), Stress-Entspannungs-Test (emotionaler, kognitiver, muskulärer Umgang mit Lärmstressoren); Hyper-, Hypo-, Normosensibilität (Chronische Stress und Erschöpfungszustände), Rhythmische Sinusarrhythmie und Herzfrequenzvariabilität (Adaptationsfähigkeit an Umweltbedingungen).
   b) Bewegung und Ernährung: Schrittzähler und Bewegungssensor (Smardwatch), Wirbelsäulendiagnostik und Flexibility-Check, Energiebilanz und Stoffwechselalter, Makronährstoffempfehlungen (in Entwicklung);
b) Prozesshafte psychobiologische Beanspruchungsmuster (als 24-h-Monitoring):
   a) Stressregulation: Chronobiologisches Monitoring (Tag/Nacht, während Arbeits- und Freizeitaktivitäten), Schlafneigungsphasen, Schlafqualität (s. Abb. 2).
   b) Psychoneuroimmunologische Verlaufs-Diagnostik, z.B. Bestimmung der Stress-Tagesrhythmik von Cortisol (Stueck, Agostini, Villegas, & Sack, 2018).

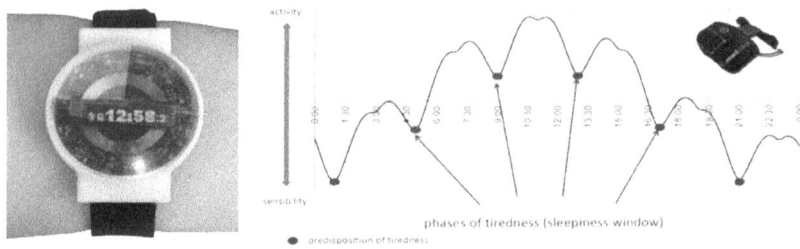

**Abbildung 2.** 24 h-Monitoring mit Biofeedback mit smardwatch-System: Feststellung der Ermüdungspunkte, Training der kognitiven, emotionalen und muskulären Entspannung.

Vorteile dieser Ebene sind, das für den Arbeitnehmer ein Belastungs-Zustand mess-, und erlebbar wird, was zu einer erhöhten Gesundheitsbereitschaft führt. Außerdem kann ein problematischer Zustand mit Biofeedback[8] am Arbeitsplatz trainiert werden.

## 2.3 Ebene 3: Analyse der Beanspruchungsfolgen infolge der Arbeitsbelastung

Bei wiederholtem Auftreten von Überlastungen (Ebene 1) und Beanspruchungszuständen (Ebene 3) ergeben sich längerfristige negative Beanspruchungsfolgen, die psychologisch getestet und bewertet werden:

a) Überforderungsreaktionen (Stueck & Thinschmidt, 2010), Fragen zur Hypersensibilität als Zeichen für beginnende Erschöpfungszustände (Balzer & Stueck, 2013) (Abb. 3). Arbeitsbezogene Verhaltens- und Erlebensmuster (AVEM; Schaarschmidt, 2006):
b) Spezielle Beanspruchungsfolgen, z.b. Fahrerverhalten (Zielgruppe Berufskraftfahrer).
c) Stressantreiber und konstitutionelle Besonderheiten (Chronotyp), Kontrollüberzeugungen (internal/external), Dysfunktionale stressrelevante Einstellungen, Messung „verdeckter" Einstellungen zu unterschiedlichen Gesundheits-aspekten mit Repertory Grid Technik (z.B. Zielgruppe Manager, s. Fußnote 4).

---

8   Klienten erhalten mittels der Messuhr (Abb. 2) Rückmeldungen über Muskelspannung (Elektromyogramm, Verhalten), kognitive (Hautpotenzial, Denken) und emotionelle Reaktionen (Hautwiderstand) und lernen, sie zu beeinflussen. Auch die Atmung in Kopplung zum Herzschlag RSA, Sinusarrythmie, s.Artikel mobiles Gesund-heitslabor) kann am Bildschirm in einer kleinen Übung von 3 Minuten trainiert werden. Siehe auch Fußnote 15.

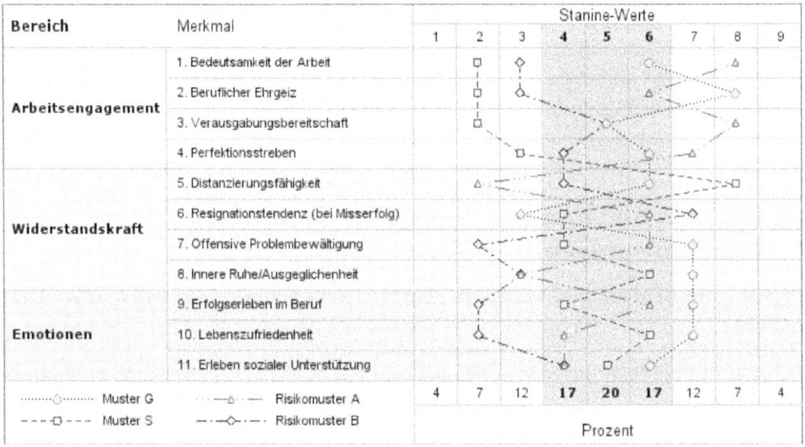

**Abbildung 3.** Primär-, Sekundärskalen und Typenbildung im AVEM.

## 2.4 Ebene 4: Messung von Ressourcen, die Gesundheit fördern

Wie die Arbeitsbelastungen (Ebene 1) als beanspruchend erlebt werden (Ebene 2 & 3) hängt von externalen Ressourcen[9] und internalen Ressourcen (Ebene 4) ab[10].

## 2.5 Ebene 5: Analyse des biozentrisch-affektiven Verhaltens

Dieser Bereich ist durch Stueck, Villegas und Toro (2010) neu entwickelt worden für das Betriebliche Gesundheitsmanagement[11] und basiert auf Arbeiten von Maturana (2011), Maturana und Varela (1980), Maturana und Verden-Zöller (2008), Toro (2002a, 2002b, 2010) und ist Voraussetzung für die Entwicklung von Gesundheitsbereitschaft bzw. für Selbstfürsorge. In diesem Bereich werden die gesunden Beziehungs-Anteile eines Menschen in 3 Aspekten diagnostiziert und gefördert (sog. Pinguin-Muster als Grundlage des Menschseins[12]; Stueck, 2018).

---

9 Umweltbedingungen, z.B. Führungsqualität, Konzeption der Arbeit, Wissen über BGM, Arbeitsschutz.
10 u.a. (a) Alter, Resilienz und Sence of Coherence, Soziale Unterstützung, Wohlbefinden, Persönlichkeit, Beziehungs-typ, Elterliche Erziehungsstile, Spirituelle Gesundheit (b) Bewältigungsaktivitäten, wie externales und internales Coping (u.a. Ärger-Ausdrucksstile) c) Einstellungen bzgl. Ernährung, Bewegung, Abhängigkeit
11 Das BGM wird hier zum Biozentrischen Betrieblichen Gesundheitsmanagement (BBGM) erweitert.
12 Symbole für Beziehungs- und Inhaltsaspekt, Empathiemodell Stueck (2013), basierend auf Maturana/Toro Arbeiten

a) Beziehung zur eigenen Person (u.a. Selbstrespekt, Selbstfürsorge, Liebesfähigkeit zu mir, Gesundheitsbedürfnisse, Entspannungsfähigkeit, Selbstwertgefühl)
b) Beziehung zu anderen: u.a. Empathie, Vertrauen, Affektive Intelligenz, Beziehungs- und Kommunikationsmuster, Toleranzfähigkeit)
c) Beziehung zur Natur: u.a. gesundes Umweltbewusstsein.

## 2.6 Ebene 6: Ableiten von Verhaltens- und Verhältnispräventiven Maßnahmen

Für alle Unternehmen werden apriori Basis-Interventionen empfohlen (ohne Diagnostik):

a) Kommunikationsmodelle (*School of Empathy*; Stueck, 2010a; Stueck, Villegas, & Toro, 2013),
b) Stressreduktionsmethoden (*School of Presence & Relaxation*; Stueck, 2007, 2010a, 2015, 2016, 2018),
c) Nonverbales Ausdrucksverhalten und Beziehungsfähigkeit (*School of Life & Trust*; Stueck & Villegas, 2008).

Folgende Spezifische diagnosegeleitete Interventionen können unter Zuhilfenahme des Masterplans „Gesunde Bildung" (Stueck, 2010c)[13] abgeleitet werden:

a) diagnosegeleitete Veränderungen bzgl. Bedingungen (Verhältnisprävention),
b) reflexive und emotionsregulierende Verhaltensänderungen (Verhaltensprävention), u.a. Supervisionen, Training von emotionsregulierenden Fähigkeiten u.a.:
   1) **Stressregulation:** HRV-Biofeedback-Training[14], Training der Ultradianen Heilreaktion (U-H-R)[15], z.B. mittels Power-Nap (Kurzschlaf) oder Selbsthypnose,
   2) **Ernährung und Bewegung:** Diagnosegeleitete Bewegungs- und Ernährungsempfehlungen (u.a. Laufband am Arbeitsplatz)

---

13 7 Bereiche sollten berücksichtigt werden: Verhaltensprävention = Präsente, Entspannte und empathische Arbeitshaltung, Supervision, Fähigkeiten, Verhältnisprävention = Konzept, Rahmenbedingungen (s. Abb.5).
14 Verfahren in der Verhaltensmedizin. Die Klienten erhalten dabei Rückmeldung über normalerweise unbewusst ablaufende Prozesse im Körper und sollen lernen, sie zu beeinflussen. Im mobilen Gesundheitslabor werden u.a. das optimale Verhältnis zwischen Atmung und Herzschlag (4:1) trainiert. Auch die muskuläre, kognitive und emotionale Entspannungsfähigkeit mittels SMARD-Watch wird erfasst und trainiert (Balzer, 2008).
15 U-H-R (Rossi, zit. In Balzer, Stueck, 2019) beschreibt einen chronobiologischen autoregulativen emotionell vegetativen Rhythmus (Hautwiderstand) mit 30% Deaktivierung und 70% Aktivierungsmustern (120 Min.), auch mit Brain-Light-Entspannungssystem, Gefäßtraining mit Mikrozirkulationsmatte trainierbar.

Der Gesundheitswürfel 99

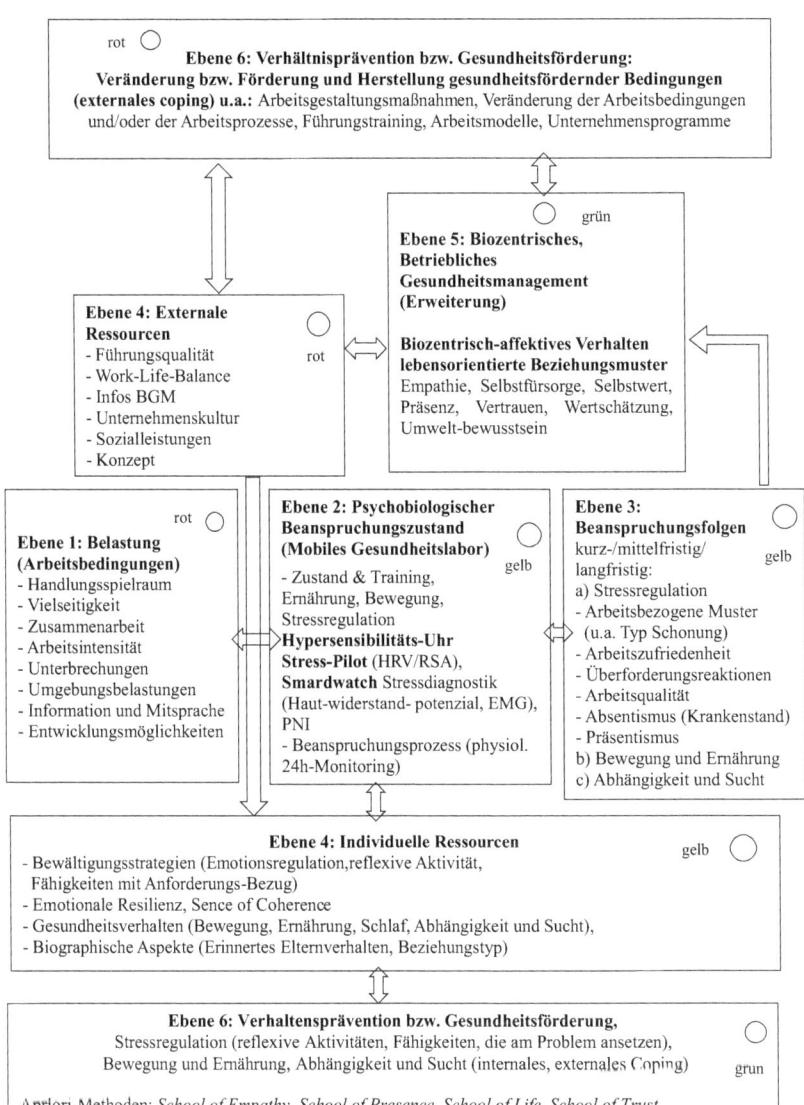

**Abbildung 4.** Gesundheitswürfel zur Auswahl der Analyse Ebenen und Befund-Darstellung; Normbasiertes Ampelsystem (Beispiel, grün = i.O., gelb = Intervention mit Zeit, rot = dringender Bedarf)

3) **Bewegung:** Bewegungs-Konzentrationstraining, für Rückengerechtes Arbeiten[16].

4) **Suchtprävention:** Info- und Trainingsangebot „Abhängigkeit" (Stueck, 2019b)

Im Schema (Abb. 4) sind die 6 Analyse-Ebenen des Gesundheitswürfels zusammengefasst. Es dient zur Planung der Gefährdungsanalyse und der Befunddarstellung.

## 3 Ablauf der Gefährdungsbeurteilung mit dem Gesundheitswürfel

Die Gefährdungsbeurteilung sollte alle 3 Jahre in folgenden 6 Schritten (PEDALE) erfolgen:

1) **Planung:** Mit Geschäftsleitung, Arbeitssicherheits- und Gesundheitsbeauftragtem werden die Bereiche (Abb. 4) festgelegt und entschieden ob der Gesundheitswürfel als Fragebogen oder Workshop mit anderem Ablauf (Stueck, 2019a, 2019b, 2019c) durchgeführt wird. Die Auftakt-Veranstaltung („Kick-off") könnte ein Gesundheitstag sein.

2) **Erhebung:** Der Kurzfragebogen (ca. 4 Seiten) ist für alle Mitarbeiter obligatorisch (Belastung und Arbeitsbedingungen, Beanspruchungsfolgen und Ressourcen). Fakultativ sind Messungen mit Laborkomponenten. Diejenigen, die mehr erfahren wollen, können die komplette Gesundheitswürfel-Version (Ebenen 1–6, ca. 6 Seiten) ausfüllen (Rücklauf 30–40%). Alle Erhebungen sind anonymisiert.

3) **Dateneingabe- und Auswertung:** alle Fragebögen werden in das Statistikprogramm SPSS eingepflegt und ausgewertet (mittels Deskriptive und Inferenzstatistik).

4) **Auswertung und Beratung für Mitarbeiter:** Es werden persönliche Gesprächstermine vereinbart. Zu diesen Terminen können zusätzliche Messungen im Labor erfolgen und persönliche Ziele vereinbart werden.

5) **Leitungsgespräch:** Es werden die Befunde zu den Ebenen 1–5 (Abb. 4, mit Ampelsystem) besprochen und Ableitungen zu Präventionsmaßnahmen mit Zielvereinbarungen vorgenommen (Abb. 5). Mit Hilfe der Abb. 5 wird geprüft, ob die Balance zwischen dem Beziehungs – und Inhaltsaspekt in den Gates (Analyse, Information, Training, Experte) und Areas (Inhalte gesunder Bildungsprozesse; Stueck, 2010c; Fußnote 14, rechte Spalte Abb. 5) berücksichtigt wurden (Pinguin-Eisbärtest; Stueck, 2018).

6) **Endbericht – und Zertifizierung:** Aufgrund aller Informationen aus allen Ebenen wird ein endgültiger anonymisierter Abschlussbericht erstellt. Es werden ein Zertifikat und Schild (z.B. Entspannte Einrichtung des BGM) verliehen.

---

16 Yoga auf dem Stuhl (Stueck, 2010), Rücken-Muskulatur-Training/Stimulationsgerät ist in Entwicklung.

Tabelle 1. Gesundheitswürfel zur diagnosegeleiteten Festlegung der Interventionen.

| Arbeitsgesundheit Themen | Gesundheitswürfel Handlungsfelder (Beziehung/Inhalt) | | Intervention Bereiche (Areas) |
|---|---|---|---|
| Ebene 1 Rahmen Bedingun-gen (rot) | | | Präsenz, Biozentrik, Spirituelle, Gesundheit, Erlebnis |
| Ebene 1 Bedin-gungen / Konzept (grün) | Workshop School of Relaxation | Anfrage Stress- reduktion | Gesunde, Lebensstile, Entspannung, Ernährung, Bewegung, Sucht (gelb) |
| Ebene 2 Biologische Bean-spruchung (gelb) | Workshop School of Empathy | | Empathie, Selbstfürsorge, Liebesfähigkeit |
| Ebene 3 Bean-spruchungs-folgen (gelb) | | | Reflexion Supervision |
| Ebene 4 Externe Ressourcen (rot) | Führungs-stärke, Mit-arbeitermoti-vation, Leitung | | Fähigkeiten Kompetenzen (gelb) |
| Ebene 4 Individuelle Ressourcen (grün & gelb) | | | Arbeits-Konzept Pädagogisches Konzept |
| Ebene 5 Biozentrik Selbstfür-sorge (grün) | Infos Bgm | Lärm-dämmung | Rahmenbedin-gungen Verhältnisprä-vention (rot) |
| Interven-tions-zugänge | **Analyse** In welchen Bereichen gibt es Probleme? | **Info** Ich möchte Gesund-heitsinfor-mationen z.B. Fachtage | **Verän-derung** **Training** Ich möchte ein Training z.B. Stress-Reduktion | **Experte** Ich möchte eine Ausbil-dung als Experte z.B. Stressreduk-tion | **Apriori Interventionen** Biozentrisch, ohne Diagnose *School of Empathy School of Relaxation/ Presence School of Trust School of Life* |

## 4 Zusammenfassung und abschließende Diskussion

Mit dem Gesundheitswürfel wurde ein Verfahren entwickelt, mit welchem modularisiert und je nach Fragestellung hinsichtlich der Bereiche: belastende Arbeitsbedingungen (Ebene 1), Beanspruchungszustand (Ebene 2), Beanspruchungsfolgen (Ebene 3), Individuelle und externale Ressourcen (Ebene 4), dem biozentrisch Affektiven Agieren (Ebene 5) und der Ableitung von Maßnahmen der Verhaltens-Verhältnisprävention (Ebene 6) eine psychische Gefährdungsanalyse durchgeführt werden kann. Durch die Normwerte können mit Hilfe eines Ampelsystems genaue Einschätzungen der Güte des Betrieblichen Gesundheit-Managements einer Institution vorgenommen werden, nicht nur bedingungs- sondern auch verhaltensseitig.

**Welche Vorteile hat die Durchführung der Gefährdungsbeurteilung psychischer Belastungen für Unternehmen?** (1) Verbesserung der Arbeitgeber-Marke, da für die Gesundheit etwas getan wird. (2) Erfüllung gesundheitsrelevanter gesetzlicher Auflagen (3) Demographischer Gesundheits-Faktor, da Mitarbeiter immer älter werden (4) eine höhere Produktivität für das Unternehmen und damit auch einen größeren Gewinn durch gesunde Mitarbeiter.

**Warum wurde das Würfelmodell gewählt?** Die sechsflächige Würfelform wurde gewählt, da man mit einem Würfel sinnlich-ästhetisch, z.B. in einer Gruppenarbeit hantieren kann, aber auch hineintreten kann – z.B. zu Gesundheitstagen- oder Messen oder ihn in die Tasche stecken kann (Biofeedback-Würfel). Zweitens geben die sechs Flächen eines Würfels keine Priorisierung der einzelnen AnalyseEbenen untereinander vor.

**In welchen Situationen ist der Gesundheitswürfel einsetzbar?** (1) Einzel- oder Gruppenarbeit, z.B. Supervisionen, Beratungsgespräche mit Leitung und Mitarbeitern, Gesundheitstage (Aufbau des mobilen Gesundheitslabors, Impulsvorträge); (2) Fragebogen-Version: Lang- und Kurzform (Papierversion, Computerwebbasiert); (3) Prä-Posttest-Evaluationen von BGM-Maßnahmen; (4) Biofeedback Würfel (Taschenversion).

**Mit welchen Zielgruppen bzw. Wo kann der Gesundheitswürfel eingesetzt werden?** Der Gesundheitswürfel ist für viele Zielgruppen einsetzbar, u.a. Lehrer, Helfer in Krisengebieten, Professionelle Fahrer, Manager, Leistungs-Sportler, Flughafen-Mitarbeiter, Pflegeeinrichtungen, Krankenhauspersonal. Die 6 Ebenen müssen je nach Zielgruppe entsprechend angepasst bzw. mit standardisierten Messverfahren „aufgefüllt" werden. Zurzeit laufen Einsätze mit adaptierten Gesundheitswürfel-Versionen im Iran (Professionelle Fahrer), Indonesien (Betriebe in Java), Deutschland (DPFA-Akademiegruppe, Lehrer und ErzieherInnen).

**Welche Vorgeschichte hat der Gesundheitswürfel?** Dieses Instrument wurde, beginnend mit den Forschungen zu Menschen in Extremsituationen (Stueck, Balzer, Hecht, Schröder, & Rigotti, 2005; Stueck & Schröder, 1995) und Lehrerbelastungen seit den 1990er bzw. 2000er Jahren an der Universität Leipzig entwickelt (Stueck, 2007, 2010a, 2010b, 2010c, 2010d, 2011b, 2013; Stueck &

Sonntag, 2005; Stueck, Rigotti, & Balzer, 2005; Stueck et al., 2005; Stueck & Trapp, 2006). In den letzten Jahren wurde das Instrumentarium beständig erweitert. Seit 2012 wurden an der DPFA-Hochschule Sachsen vor allem Laborforschungen zu verschiedenen Fragestellungen der Physiologie und Psychoneuroimmunologie in Zusammenhang mit Stress durchgeführt (Mueller, Stueck, & Balzer, 2014) und in der Praxis angewendet, v.a. im Erzieherinnenbereich für die Diagnostik der Bereiche (Birke et al., 2018), u.a. mit einer Farbdiagnostik. Ausserdem wurden die psychischen Dimensionen mit hormonellen Besonderheiten bzw. mit dem physiologischen Parameter der Hypersensibilität der Haut korreliert. 2019 wurden eine Reihe von internationalen Praxiserprobungen mit Studien durchgeführt bzw. werden vorbereitet: mit Berufskraftfahrern im Iran (Stueck, 2019; Stueck et al., 2019) und mit Mitarbeitern einer Indonesischen Reederei in Indonesien (Stueck, Mulyati, & Utami, 2019). Außerdem wird seit 2018 der Gesundheitswürfel für die Schulen der DPFA-Akademiegruppe verwendet. Der Gesundheitswürfel wurde seit den Forschungen zum Kinderyoga (Stueck, 1997) auch zur psychischen Gefährdungsbeurteilung für Kinder entwickelt und wird in einem gesonderten Artikel beschrieben.

## 5 Affiliation

Prof. Dr. Marcus Stueck (Entwickler GH-Würfel, Head of Research)
Institution: DPFA-Akademie für Arbeitsgesundheit / International Research Academy-Bionet Leipzig.
Address: DPFA-Akademie für Arbeitsgesundheit, Täubchenweg 83, 04317 Leipzig, Germany.
E-mail: marcus.stueck@dpfa-hs.de

## 6 Referenzliste

Balzer, H.-U., & Stueck, M. (2019). *Einführung in die Chronopsychobiologie*. Manuscript submitted for publication.

Birke, A., Rieche, A., Wittwer, C., Zschocke, N., Hamann, L., Knoche, V., ... Stueck, M. (2018). *Die Anwendungen des Gesundheitswürfels im Erzieherbereich. Psychologische, Physiologische und Psychoneuroimmunologische Effektbestimmung*. Unpublished manuscript, International Research Academy-Bionet, Leipzig.

Maturana, H. (2011). *Die Biologie der Realität*. Berlin: Suhrkamp Verlag.

Maturana, H., & Francisco, V. (1984). *Der Baum der Erkenntnis. Die biologischen Wurzeln menschlichen Erkennens*. Frankfurt am Main: Deutsche Übersetzung von Kurt Ludewig.

Maturana, H., & Varela, F. (1980). *Autopoesis and Cognition. The Realization of the Living*. Kluver: Language of Science.

Maturana, M., & Verden-Zöller, G. (2008). *The Origin of Humanness in the Biology of Love*. Exeter: Imprint Academic.

Molnar, M., Geißler-Gruber, B., & Haiden, C. (2011). Betriebliche Analyse der Arbeitsbedingungen. In WKÖ, ÖGB (Hrsg.), *IMPULS-Broschüre und IMPULS-Test* (S. 1–54). Wien: Europäischen Agentur für Sicherheit und Gesundheitsschutz am Arbeitsplatz.

Mueller, S., Stueck, M., & Balzer, H.-U. (2014). Zusammenhang von Biografie, Stress & Körperreaktionen bei Erziehern: Psycho-physiologische Laboruntersuchungen zur Erziehergesundheit. *ErgoMed Praktische Arbeitsmedizin*, (6), 24–30.

Prochaska, J. O., & DiClemente, C. C. (1982). Transtheoretical therapy: Toward a more integrative change model. *Psychotherapy: Theory, Research, Practice, 19*(3), 276–288.

Rudow, B. (2001). *Psychische Belastungen im Lehrerberuf.* GUV-I 8760 Beurteilung von Gefährdungen und Belastungen an Lehrerarbeitsplätzen, München.

Schaarschmidt, U. (2006). AVEM - ein persönlichkeitsdiagnostisches Instrument für die berufsbezogene Rehabilitation. In Arbeitskreis Klinische Psychologie in der Rehabilitation BDP (Hrsg.), *Psychologische Diagnostik - Weichenstellung für den Reha-Verlauf* (S. 59–82). Bonn: Deutscher Psychologen Verlag GmbH.

Stueck, M. (1997). *Wie man Belastungen abbauen kann. Das Entspannungstraining mit Yogaelementen für Kinder*. Strasburg: Schibri.

Stueck, M. (2007). *Neue Wege: Yoga und Biodanza in der Stressreduktion für Lehrer* (Habilitation). Universität Leipzig, Leipzig.

Stueck, M. (2010a). *Stressreduktion mit Yogaelementen für belastete Berufsfelder (School of Presence & Relaxation)*. Strassburg: Schibri.

Stueck, M. (2010b). *Systemische biozentrische Diagnostik für den Lehrerberuf: Der Gesundheitswürfel*. Leipzig: Penguin & Polar Bear Edition.

Stueck, M. (2010c). *Forscher, Künstler, Konstrukteure. Frühe Bildung auf dem Prüfstand*. Strassburg: Schibri.

Stueck, M. (2010d). Yoga auf dem Stuhl. In M. Thinschmidt (Hrsg.), *Handbuch für ErzieherInnengesundheit* (S.134). Dresden: Ministerium für Kultus und Soziales.

Stueck, M. (2011a). *Risikoanalyse-Instrument für Belastungen bei Kindern und Jugendlichen*. Unpublished manuscript, International Research Academy – Bionet, Leipzig.

Stueck, M. (2011b). *Risikoanalyse-Instrument für Belastungen bei Lehrern und Erzieherinnen zur Erstellung von Arbeitsanalysen*. Unpublished manuscript, International Research Academy – Bionet, Leipzig.

Stueck, M. (2013a). Die Grundlagen einer Theorie von sich selbstorganisierenden empathischen Netzwerken: Historische Ursprünge. In E. Witruk & A. Wilcke (Hrsg.), *Beiträge zur Pädagogischen und Rehabilitationspsychologie, Band 4: Historical and Cross-Cultural Aspects of Psychology* (S. 131–140). Frankfurt am Main: Peter Lang.

Stueck, M. (2013b). School of Empathy: Introduction and first results. In E. Witruk & A. Wilcke (Hrsg.), *Beiträge zur Pädagogischen und Rehabilitationspsychologie, Band 4: Historical and Cross-Cultural Aspects of Psychology* (S. 497–510). Frankfurt am Main: Peter Lang.

Stueck, M. (2015). Biodanza – Inklusion geht nur mit geschlossenen Augen! *Praxishandbuch Kinder unter 3, Ausgabe 14*, 1, 1–10.

Stueck, M. (2016). Ten Steps of Stress Reduction: The Intercultural Adapted Version of Training of Stress Reduction with Elements of Relaxation (STRAIMY®-International). In E. Witruk, S. Novita, Y. Lee, & D. S. Utami, *Studies of Educational and Rehabilitation Psychology, vol. 7: Dyslexia and traumatic experiences* (pp. 163–170). Frankfurt am Main: Peter Lang.

Stueck, M. (2018). How Polar Bears and Penguins got together. Fundamentals of a School of Empathy and Complete Science. In M. E. Murueta, E. Galindo, & M. Stueck. *Diálogo Europeo-Latnoamericano sobre Transformación Educativa 1* (pp. 31–46). Mexico City: Edición Amapsi Editorial.

Stueck, M. (2019a). *Der Gesundheitswürfel als Workshop*. Leipzig: Penguin & Polar Bear Edition.

Stueck, M. (2019b). *Infos zur Abhängigkeit*. Unpublished manuscript, International Research Academy-Bionet, Leipzig.

Stueck, M. (2019c). *The Health Cube for drivers*. Manuscript submitted for publication.

Stueck, M., & Balzer, H.-U. (2019). *Die physiologische und psychologische Erfassung der Hypersensibilität*. Manuscript submitted for publication.

Stueck, M., & Schröder, H. (1995). *Erfolgsdruck lastete auf der Aconcagua Expedition*. Wissenschaftsteil der Leipziger Volkszeitung (S. 12), Leipzig.

Stueck, M., & Sonntag, A. (2005). Normativ auffälliges Beanspruchungserleben bei Lehrern. *ErgoMed Praktische Arbeitsmedizin, 29*(4), 105–113.

Stueck, M., & Thinschmidt, M. (2010). Analyse-Fragebogen zur Feststellung von Belastungen im ErzieherInnenberuf. In M. Thinschmidt (Hrsg.), *Handbuch für ErzieherInnengesundheit* (S.125). Dresden: Ministerium für Kultus und Soziales.

Stueck, M., & Trapp, S. (2006). Belastungserleben und Problembewältigung bei Sozialpädagogischen PraktikerInnen. *ErgoMed Praktische Arbeitsmedizin, 30*(4), 116–126.

Stueck, M., & Villegas, A. (2008). *Zur Gesundheit tanzen*. Strassburg: Schibri.

Stueck, M., Agostini, S., Villegas, A., & Sack, U. (2018, October). *Pre-Post-Effekte im Tagesverlauf von Cortisol*. Paper session presented at the European Biodanza Congress, Sevilla, Spain.

Stueck, M., Balzer, H. U., Hecht, K., Schröder, H., & Rigotti, T. (2005). Psychological and Psychophysiological effects of a High Mountains Expedition to Tibet. *Journal of Human Performance in Extreme Environments, 8*(1), 11–20.

Stueck, M., Balzer, H.-U., Mueller S., & Sack, U. (2019). Das Mobile Gesundheitslabor - Ein Bestandteil des Gesundheitswürfels zur Psychischen Gefährdungs- und Ressourcenbeurteilung im Rahmen des Biozentrischen und Betrieblichen Gesundheitsmanagements (BGM) in Unternehmen und Institutionen. In E. Witruk & D. S. Utami, *Educational and Rehabilitation Psychology (vol. 8): Traumatic experiences and dyslexia*. Manuscript submitted for publication.

Stueck, M., Delshad, V., Roudini, J., Balzer, H.-U., & Sack, U. (2019). *The Health Cube and its application with Iranian drivers*. Manuscript submitted for publication.

Stueck, M., Delshad, V., Roudini, J., Khankeh, H., Ranjbar, M., Reschke, K., ... Sack, U. (2019). *Health Cube with School of Empathy and Stress reduction for Iranian Drivers New tools for Traffic Psychology & Biocentric Health Management in Iran*. Manuscript submitted for publication.

Stueck, M., Mulyati, R., & Utami, D. S. (2019). *Health Cube and AVEM*. Unpublished manuscript, International Research Academy-Bionet, Leipzig.

Stueck, M., Neumann, D., Mayer, L., Rillich, K., Dobrig, P., Lahm, B., ...Wallenhauer, P. (2010). Psychologische Präventionsansätze in Handlungsfeldern der sozialen Arbeit. In E. Witruk (Hrsg.), *Beiträge zur Pädagogischen und Rehabilitationspsychologie. Learning, Adjustment and Stress Disorders* (S. 343–358). Frankfurt am Main: Peter Lang.

Stueck, M., Rigotti, T., & Balzer, U. (2005). Wie reagieren Lehrer bei Belastungen? Berufliche Bewältigungsmuster und psychophysiologische Korrelate. *Psychologie in Erziehung und Unterricht, 52*(4), 250–260.

Stueck, M., Schoppe, S., Lahn, F., & Toro, R. (2013). Was nützt es sich in jemanden hineinzuversetzen, ohne zu handeln? *ErgoMed Praktische Arbeitsmedizin, 6*(37), 38–46.

Stueck, M., Villegas, A., & Toro R. (2013). *Nonverbale Aspekte wertschätzender Kommunikation in Kindertagesstätten*. Strassburg: Schibri.

Stueck, M., Villegas, A., & Toro, R. (2010). *Nonverbale Aspekte Wertschätzender Kommunikation in Kindertagesstätten: Empathieschule für Pädagogen. Beiträge zur Bildungsgesundheit, Band 8*. Strasburg: Schibri-Verlag.

Toro, R. (2002a). *Das Biozentrische Prinzip*. Unpublished manuscript, Biodanza School Leipzig, Germany.

Toro, R. (2002b). *Biozentrische Erziehung*. Unpublished manuscript, Biodanza School Leipzig, Germany.

Toro, R. (2010). *Das System Biodanza*. Hannover: Tinto-Verlag.

I. P. R. Chathuranga, Buddhiphraba D. D. Pathirana, & Marcus Stueck

# Cultural Adaptation of Biodanza to Manage Stress within Sri Lankan Youth and Adolescence

**Abstract:** Biodanza is a route of body movements; combined with music applied to enhance the positive feelings of the participants. It is successfully utilised for developing the health and well-being of target groups across the globe. Biodanza is directly addressing and reinforces intraindividual and interindividual resources by reducing high-stress levels of the affected people. As adolescents continuously experience a myriad of social, emotional, commercial and cultural issues, especially those from the developing world in their struggle to achieve life targets. However, the failures of achieving them may lead to various concerns and frustrations. However, due to resource constraints, counselling and therapeutic services may not be available to youth adolescents living in the developing world including Sri Lanka. Thus, Biodanza can be described as a novel approach which positively addresses youth and adolescent issues. However, the concept of Biodanza is an unknown word in many developing countries including Sri Lanka. Further, when using Biodanza for stress alleviation among Sri Lankan adolescence; the original content of Biodanza may not ideally fit into the collective culture and local attitudes. Therefore, the present study explored using a cultural adapted form of Biodanza to reduce stress within Sri Lankan adolescence. The participants were 30 adolescents between 15 to 20 years, selected through convenient sampling. The theme used was a familiar folktale of a village chieftain visiting heaven on a flying elephant. The participant's pre and post-stress levels were measured using a survey questionnaire. Paired sample t-test conveyed that there is a significant reduction of stress after the Biodanza. The study discusses the cultural adaptation of Biodanza for Sri Lankan youth and adolescence and provides recommendations to Sri Lankan policy makers, counsellors and educationists.

**Keywords:** Biodanza, stress management, Sri Lanka, adolescence, culture

## 1 Introduction

Biodanza was initially created by Rolando Toro (1995). It can be described as a systematic approach which has spread to 54 countries, developed as well as developing. Research carried out on Biodanza conveys its effectiveness of stress alleviation across gender, varied age groups and countries. Unfortunately, extremely few systematic studies of Biodanza are recorded for Sri Lanka (Pathirana & Stueck, 2017).

On the other hand, Sri Lankan youth and adolescents have reported experiencing very high levels of stress. It could be due to the exam pressure of being exposed to competitive educations as well as natural/man/made disasters that the country collectively underwent. However, resources and service provision constraints prevent them from having access to therapeutic and counselling services which those in developed countries are privileged of having. Therefore, Bodanza may serve as an economically feasible intervention to reduce stress and other related problems of Sri Lankan adolescence. However, using Biodanza requires to be carried out cautiously due to its Western components which heavily emphasise on touching the participants during the sessions. It was envisaged that Sri Lankan adolescents might not positively respond to these aspects as well as Western themes if they were to be mirrored. Thus, the main objective of the present study was to explore whether using Biodanza with the culturally sensitive theme would reduce stress within Sri Lankan adolescence.

## 2 Theoretical Review

Biodanza can be described as a contemporary intervention to promote health and well-being. It aims to work with dance and group experiences to reinforce intraindividual and interindividual resources, reduce stress and intends to encourage self-regulation (Toro, 1995) within individuals. The name, 'Biodanza' was a neologism from the Greek "bio" (life) and the Spanish "Danza" (dance), to convey the meaning 'the dance of life' (Stueck & Tofts, 2016). It has been described as a systematic method of self-development which deepens self-awareness through music, body movements and positive feelings (Stueck, 2011). It also seeks to promote the ability to make a holistic link to self, emotions as well as expressing them to deepen the bonds with others (Stueck, 2004).

Rolando Toro (1995) developed the theoretical model of Biodanza. According to Toro (1995), Biodanza aims to encourage psychophysiological self-organization (self-regulation) and mobilise self-healing. Thus, compared to Western Psychotherapeutics which heavily concentrates on the cause or the problems of Biodanza leans on a person's hidden potential and available resources (Toro, 1995).

An official definition of Biodanza is given by the International Biocentric Foundation (2005) as a human integration system of organic renewal, of affective re-education while re-learning original functions of life. Their definition contains five keywords; there are human integration, organic renewal, affective re-education, re-learning of life original functions, integrative "Vivencias" (being here and now).

Empirical Biodanza research was initiated in the 1990s. A Germen-Argentinian research group in Argentina undertook the first classic empirical study on stress, well-being and Biodanza (Stueck et al., 2009). In 2008, Stueck and Villegas developed a master plan of Biodanza research which contained eight aspects. In a study carried out to explore the Biodanza on first graders by Stueck, Villegas, Schoenichen, Bauer, Tofts, and Sack (2013), they found that there was a statistically significant improvement in emotion regulation outcomes, prosocial and internalising behavior among the experimental group in comparison to the controls. Studies carried out on Biodanza also convey that it may create physiological changes in participants leading to a sense of well-being, self-acceptance, positive relations, and environmental control (Stueck, 2009) while promoting.

Stress is a clear risk factor for mental health difficulties, which have been estimated to affect approximately one in five children ages 9 to 17 years (U.S. Department of Health and Human Services, 1999), especially for adolescents as they are going through a developmental trajectory which creates stress due to physiological as well as psychological issues. Research convey that academic stress may happen due to varied sources, such as interpersonal, intrapersonal, academic, and environmental issues (Ross, Niebling, Bradley & Heckert, 1999) and may cause change in sleep habits, vacations and breaks, change in eating habits, increased workload and new responsibilities (Ross et al., 1999). Literature conveys that high levels of academic achievements may generate high levels of stress among adolescents and youth (Suldo, Shaunessy, & Hardesty, 2008).

The findings from present research may be further used to examine which sources of stress cause the highest levels of stress among students, and these results also help to create stress management programs.

Perceptions of academic stress and coping strategies might differ across cultures. Hence, cultural variations of its aetiology require to be understood before developing suitable interventions (Misran & Castillo, 2004). Studies on stress carried out in the Sri Lankan milieu convey that Sri Lankan youth, adolescents and children display high levels of stress due to conflict, natural disasters as well as daily stressors (Miller, Fernando, & Berger, 2009). However, very few studies have addressed using interventions such as Biodanza with Sri Lankan youth have ((Pathirana & Stueck, 2017).

Among multitude to stress management strategies, research reports dance to be an innovative and successful form. For example, Jeong, Hong, Lee, Park & Suh (2005) found 12 weeks of dance movement therapy improved the psychological health of adolescents with mild depression.

While recognising the importance of empirical research on stress and stress management about Sri Lankan adolescents, the outcome of the present research also points to the need of policies and interventions that focus on reducing proximal daily stressors that are silent to Sri Lankan adolescents/youth.

# 3 Method

## 3.1 Participants

Thirty-eight participants enrolled to participate in the Biodanza workshop. However, only 30 people (22 females and eight males) completed the workshop, comprising of two phases. The participants were between 15 to 25 years ($M = 16.43$; $SD = 1.331$). All participants were Sinhala Buddhists with twenty-two (73.3%) living in villages and 8 (26.7%) in cities.

## 3.2 Measurement Tools

### 3.2.1 Questionnaire

A self-reported survey questionnaire was used to measure participants' levels of stress before and after the Biodanza interventions. The questionnaire was divided into two sections. Section I aimed to gather the demographic information (e.g., age, gender, grade) of the participants, while section II evaluated the levels of stress ($n = 20$ statements) within the participants with a rating scale in a range of "strongly agree" to "strongly disagree".

### 3.2.2 Folktale

The story of the Village Cheftian's (Chilef of the the village) Journey to Heaven:

> 'Once upon a time in a faraway village in Sri Lanka lived a village cheftian One day on his way home after the new year festival in his village, he sees a beautiful white elephant flying from the sky and eating sugar cane in his land. He hides and waits till the elephant finish eating. He grabs the tail of the elephant when the elephant is about to fly away. The elephant flies to heaven and the cheftian sees and experiences many wonders. When the elephant flies back the cheftian grab the tail of the elephant and arrive in his village. The next day, the cheftian describe to his family, friends and relatives his experience. They too want to visit the heaven. Thus, on the next night, a retinue of villagers hide and wait for the elephant and arrive from heaven. They too see many wonders. Among them is 'Kapruka' (A wishing tree which fulfils the wishes of the requestors). The villagers wish for things they want, arrive in their village and live happily ever after.'

### 3.2.3 Music

Biodanza uses music, movement and positive feelings to deepen self-awareness. Therefore, dancing movements and music play an important role in it. The present research used three Sri Lankan instrumental music tracks of Sinhalese songs to avid distractions that the lyrics may have on the participants. The intention of using music was to focus participants' attention on their internal emotions, feelings and imaginations.

## 4 Results

The present study aimed to explore the impact of Biodanza in reducing the stress levels of Sri Lankan students with a selected group from the University of Peradeniya. Paired sample t-test on SPSS was conducted to evaluate whether being exposed to Biodanza affected the stress levels of the participants'. As depicted in Figure 1, results conveyed that there is statistically significant difference between pre-test ($M = 50.2$, $SD = 11.66$) and post-test ($M = 42.6$, $SD = 12.63$) conditions: $t(29) = 3.951$, $p = 0.0004$.

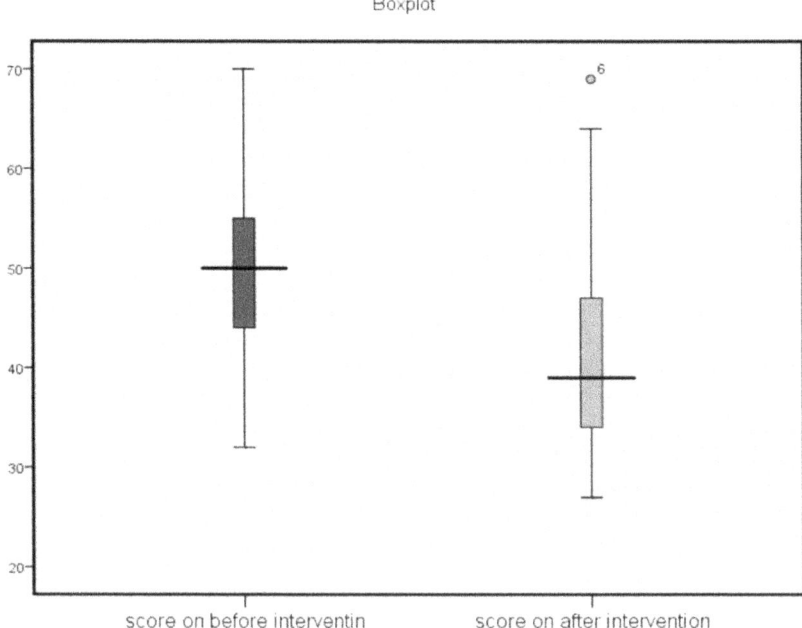

Figure 1. Levels of stress before and after the Biodanza intervention

## 5 Discussion and Conclusion

The present study records the following limitations. First, inhibitions created due to mixed-gendered participation may have impacted the outcomes of the programs. Generally, in Sri Lankan schools, adolescents do not participate in mix-gendered activities. As this is the first time that the culturally sensitive Biodanza was applied in Sri Lankan schools, with co-participation of girls and boys; the authors envisage that co-participation may have created inhibitions and initial reluctance to participate and may have affected the group cohesiveness and thus the outcomes of the study. For instance, when the participants were provided with the opportunity to form groups; the first author observed that they often attempted to form the same gendered groups resulting more time taken to explain the activities. Therefore, it is recommended that future research requires to consider this aspect when conducting group activities with mix gendered adolescent groups, especially in school settings.

Second, the methodological limitations of the study also require to be recorded. Generally, the Biodanza research uses its efficacy through laboratory tests using sophisticated instruments to measure physiological changes of participants.

However, due to resource constraints, the present study used a pre and post-survey questionnaire. As Sri Lankan adolescents and youth were somewhat unfamiliar with consent forms and completing survey questionnaires a considerable amount of time had to be spent on explaining the reasons for using these documents.

It could be due to the limited exposure which participants may have had with training programs/workshops. Therefore, based on the outcomes of the present study; authors recommend the school going adolescents to be exposed to more co-participatory activities, training and awareness programs.

The Biodanza workshop was conducted in the dancing room of the school with teachers and some students as onlookers, at certain times. Thus, even though Biodanza principles state that all the individuals in the room have to be participants and not be onlookers; due to dancing practices held in the venue; this rule could not be strictly followed and is recorded as a limitation. Authors believe that this may also have created inhibitions as some participants displayed more confidence when onlookers were not present.

The authors adapted Biodanza intervention to Sri Lankan cultural context using a storyline which was familiar to the Sri Lankans along with Sri Lankan musical tracks. However, the present study was limited to the Sri Lankan student community. Thus, future research required to explore myriad of culturally sensitive approaches of using Biodanza for reducing stress and related issues with varied Sri Lankan communities (e.g., University students, professional groups, and individuals from challenging environments). Moreover, the authors are of the opinion that the effectiveness of Biodanza on promoting health and well-being in the Sri Lankan milieu can be more effectively analyzed using qualitative methods.

The outcomes of the present research convey that the development of a cultural-sensitive Biodanza program is a feasible practice and a promising method to promote well-being and decrease stress within Sri Lankan adolescents. The participants positively responded, and actively engaged in the activities conducted. Participants also reported that they felt comfortable with Biodanza than with traditional counselling.

# 6 Affiliations

I. P. R. Chathuranga
Institution: Department of Psychology, University of Peradeniya
Address: University of Peradeniya, Peradeniya, Sri Lanka
E-mail: cpathirana47@gmail.com

Dr. Buddhiprabha D. D. Pathirana
Institution: University of Peradeniya
Address: Head, Department of Psychology, University of Peradeniya
E-mail: buddhiprabha2001@yahoo.com

Prof. Dr. Marcus Stueck
Institution: DPFA-Academy of Work and Health / International Research Academy – BIONET
Address: DPFA-Weiterbildung GmbH, Taeubchenweg 83, 04317 Leipzig, Germany.
E-mail: marcus.stueck@dpfa-hs.de

# 7 References

Jeong, Y. J., Hong, S. C., Lee, M., Park, M. C., Kim, Y. K., & Suh, C. M. (2005). Dance/movement therapy improves emotional responses and modulates neurohormones in adolescents with mild depression. *International Journal of Neuroscience, 115*(12), 1711–1720.

Miller, K. E., Fernando, G. A., & Berger, D. E. (2009). Daily stressors in the lives of Sri Lankan Youth: A mixed method approach to assessment in a context of war and natural disaster. *War and Trauma Foundation,* 187–200.

Misran, R., & Castillo, L. G. (2004). Academic Stress among College Students: Comparison of American and International Students. *International Journal of Stress Management, 11* (2), 132–148.

Pathirana, B.D.D., & Stueck, M. (2017, September). Biodanza for stress management: A case study from Sri Lanka. Paper presented in the International Conference "Dyslexia and Traumatic Experience" Educational and Rehabilitation Psychology, University of Leipzig, Leipzig, Germany.

Ross, S., Niebling, B. C., & Heckert, T. M. (1999). Sources of stress among college students. *College Student Journal, 33*(2), 312–317.

Stueck, M. (2004). Stress management in schools: an empirical investigation of a stress management system. *Social Work Practitioner-Researcher, 16*(2), 216–230.

Stueck, M. (2011). The concept of system related to stress reduction (SYSRED) in educational fields. *Problem of Education in the 21st Century, volume 29,* 119–130.

Stueck, M., & Toftes, P. S. (2016). Biodanza effects on stress reduction and well-being – A review of study quality and outcome. *Signum Temporis,* 57–66.

Stueck, M., & Villegas A. (2008): The effects of Biodanza Extensions. In M. Stueck and A. Villegas, *Dance towards Health* (pp. 238–243). Berlin: Schibri Verlag.

Stueck, M., Villegas, A., Bauer, K., Terren, R., Toro, V., & Sack, U. (2009). Psycho-Immunological Process Evaluation of Biodanza. *Journal of Pedagogy and Psychology,* 99–113.

Stueck, M., Villegas, A., Schoenichen, C., Bauer, K., Tofts, P., & Sack, U. (2013). Effects of an evidence-based dance program (TANZPRO-Biodanza) for kindergarten children aged four to six on immunoglobulin A, testosterone and heart rate. *Problems of Education in the 21st Century, 56,* 128–143.

Suldo, S. M., Shaunessy, E., & Hardesty, R. (2008). Relationships among stress, coping, and mental health in high-achieving high school students. *Psychology in the Schools, 45*(4), 273–290. doi:10.1002/pits.20300

Toro, R. (1995). *The Theory of Biodanza*. Unpublished Material, School of Biodanza Leipzig, Leipzig. Retrieved on August 21, 2018 from http://www.biodanzaschule-leipzig.de.

U.S. Department of Health and Human Services. (1999). *Mental health: A report of the surgeon general*. Retrieved on August 4, 2018 from https://profiles.nlm.nih.gov/ps/access/NNBBHS.pdf

Edgar Galindo

# Teaching Academic, Social and Independence Skills to Slum Children

**Abstract:** This paper explains the work done with children growing up in slums in Mexico and Portugal. Some introductory considerations about factors determining psychological development are made. Development is a function of external and internal factors. Internal factors include a healthy body and external factors an environment with minimal well-being conditions, like a functioning family, a health and educational system, and social peace. Variations in internal and/or external factors can produce a developmental deviation and then developmental problems and/or disorders like intellectual disability, learning disorders, ADHD, etc. Simple, cheap, efficient and scientifically based intervention programs are urgently needed. The author applied the Applied Behavior Analysis techniques to train independence, social & academic skills to slum children with intellectual, physical or sensorial disabilities in Mexico. Similar procedures were applied to train children with school failure problems in a slum-like community in Portugal. Some results are presented regarding behavioral objectives attained by individual children in different training programs. Some cases of children with blindness, intellectual disability or school failure problems are briefly analyzed. Behavioral intervention programs were successful independently of the case, age or problem treated.

**Keywords:** Applied Behavior Analysis, children at risk, SEN children, school failure

## 1 Introduction

This paper explains the work done with children growing up in slums in Mexico and Portugal. Two types of cases are analyzed, namely, children born with a deficiency and children with relatively normal development, but having problems at school for different (sometimes unknown) reasons. Intervention procedures will be briefly explained, and some illustrative cases will be shown. Initially, some primary considerations about factors determining psychological development are necessary.

Psychological development is usually a process characterized by an increasing acquisition of diverse skills in the first years of life. If we look at the development of a newborn child, it is evident that he shows every day more complex behaviors enabling him to master new situations. Cognitive and emotional processes correlated with neurobiological transformations are at work to produce new behavioral repertoires, i.e., new skills allowing the child to solve problems and move around with independence. Growing means acquiring skills to cope with new environmental challenges. This process is especially accelerated in infancy, but it seems to proceed the whole life long, until a moment of decline, somewhere in an elderly age (see Baltes, Staudinger, & Lindenberger, 1999). Being a result of the dialectical interaction of numerous factors, psychological development is not a linear process, but it is characterized by different speeds, by different qualities and even by returns to early stages. Nevertheless, it is clear that a developing person has to master new and more complex tasks during his/her life. We can even say there are specific developmental tasks to be solved in different more or less good defined stages of human life (Mash & Wolfe, 2016). For instance, a 6–7-years-old child is expected to speak clearly, play properly with other children, go alone to the toilet, keep himself clean, control his/her emotions and move at home & school without help. If the child is not able to do so, he/she cannot go to school, and the existence of a problem is taken for granted; a psychological intervention is usually recommended. Similar observations can be done, regarding a 20, 30 or 50 years old person, only developmental tasks are different.

Now, psychological development is a result of the interaction between internal and external factors (Bijou, 1963). Internal factors are biological properties of the newborn organism, like a nervous & muscular system, a genetic endowment, senses and probably inherited vulnerabilities and reaction properties. External factors refer to the physical & social environment. A harmonic development ("normal" is probably not the right word) requires a relatively healthy body. Biological properties of the body can vary, but they must remain within certain limits to allow a sound development. The same is true for physical and social factors: They can vary, and in fact, they do vary widely from a person to other, but variations must remain within certain limits to permit a sound psychological development. This means some changes in internal and/or external factors can have negative consequences: Extreme variations in organic anomalies or/and in external conditions can limit the psychological development. Blindness, deafness, a cerebral lesion, a genetic variation, a lack of a hand, can disturb development.

Regarding physical and social factors, the absence of a minimal set of living conditions can disturb development, even in the body is healthy. Bronfenbrenner (2004) contributed to the understanding of the concept social environment: parents, family, school, friends, ethnic group, nation, social & political structures, culture are determining factors of psychological development. A child needs peaceful, stable conditions to develop properly. That is to say, child maltreatment, unstable families, violent relations, marginalisation, poverty, malnutrition, war, social violence and the lack of educational and/or medical services can disturb development. Vygotsky (see Rieber & Carton, 1993) added a critical remark: An abnormal factor (organic or environmental) affecting psychological development multiplies its adverse effects, i.e., a primary defect will give rise to secondary defects, producing tertiary defects and so on. A therapeutic intervention ("creating social bridges" says Vygotsky) is therefore essential to eliminate or at least reduce the effects of a negative factor.

On the other hand, research on development has shown an intimate dialectic relationship between internal (organic) and external factors (environmental). Since many years ago, it is taken for granted that psychological development relays on a neurological maturation process. Presently, we know the influence between environment and organism is mutual: learning requires a neural basis, but experience also influences the brain and other nervous structures (Knudsen, 2004). Moreover, the effects of experience on the nervous system are particularly strong during a limited period in child development, i.e., there are sensitive (or critical) periods in which experience seems to instruct neural structures a way of processing information. It seems that experience during a sensitive period modifies neural architecture in fundamental ways. This knowledge has dramatic consequences for our understanding of child development. On the one hand, some skills are better learned in some developmental periods, for instance, language capacities. On the other hand, good or bad experiences in a sensitive period have enduring consequences for the human being. It means injury, illness, neglect, malnutrition, maltreatment or other negative factors occurring in a sensitive period can make it difficult for a child to acquire the necessary skills to accomplish his/her developmental tasks. When this happens, the child will have more difficulties to gain those skills. It is a controversial question if it is possible that children who do not get the proper stimulation during these periods will ever gain the skills they should have gained, even if they receive a proper education or training. The same is true for bad experiences occurring in sensitive periods, is it possible to revert the negative effects through therapy? Nevertheless, it is a fact these children need help: special education, treatment, therapy or training.

## 2 Problems and Disorders

The most obvious consequence of such a deviation of development is often a disorder: autism, intellectual disability, specific learning disorders, attention deficit hyperactivity disorder (ADHD), emotional & behavior disorders. Sometimes it is not a disorder "stricto sensu", but an organic state, which under given circumstances can limit development, giving rise to a further problem, like blindness, deafness, and some childhood diseases. Scientists have created a term to refer to children, who have a higher probability of suffering mental health problems due to their organic state at birth or to their living conditions: children at risk. They are children from disadvantaged families and neighbourhoods, from abusive or neglectful families, infants receiving inadequate child care, born with very low weight, or born to parents with mental illness or substance abuse problems (Mash & Wolfe, 2016).

Other cases should be added to this list, namely, children born with sensorial deficiencies, like blindness or/and deafness, with physical disabilities and/or health impairments, like cerebral palsy, and born with genetic disorders, like Down Syndrome. These are the "exceptional children" (Heward, 2017), also called "children with special educational needs" (SEN) (Frederickson & Cline, 2015) to emphasise the pedagogical side of their problem. Last but not least, we have to add to this list those children who have a relatively "normal" development, but have difficulties in responding to school requirements, i.e., the so-called "students at risk for academic failure" (Darensbourg & Blake, 2013), or "students at risk for school failure" (Hamre & Pianta, 2005) or "children at risk for early academic problems" (McClelland, Morrison, & Holmes, 2000) or "students academically at-risk" (Sapp, 1996):

> Academically at-risk students are those who are one or more years behind their cohort group. This is particularly problematic in the areas of reading and mathematical skills. Moreover, becoming a parent, being adjudicated a delinquent, or falling behind in the number of credits earned can place a student in the at-risk category for academic failure (...) In summary, any factors that place a student at risk for school failure connote being "at-risk" (Sapp, 1996, p. 124).

This is a special group of children, due to the fact that they hardly fall into the category of SEN children, but they do have psychological problems, which must be urgently solved in order to avoid further psychosocial deviations, like behavior problems, drug abuPse, delinquency, unemployment and psychiatric disorders (Catalano, Loeber, & MacKinney, 1999; Martin, Del Barrio, Montero, Fernandez, Gutierrez, & Ochaita, 2003). This group of children seems to be very numerous. School failure has been a topic of discussion and research in the most developed countries since many years ago (Organization for Economic Co-operation and Development [OECD], 1998) and many corrective measures have been applied in Europe by educational agencies, focusing on social, educational, political and economic factors contributing to the problem. But school failure still exists as a huge challenge not only in the rich OECD countries but much more in the developing world (Mendoza, 2012). The problem is aggravated by the fact that very little applied research on the concrete needs of these children has been made because many authors prefer to describe the situation instead of looking for solutions (Wood, Frank, & Wacker, 1998). In consequence, children with school failure difficulties once identified, are often taught with the same methods that did not work in the past.

The problems of children growing up in slums must be understood in this context. Living in poverty conditions is a risk factor. Research on children in poverty in the United States shows they are more than other children exposed to factors that may impair brain development, affecting psychological development (Huffman, Mehlinger, & Kerivan, 2000; Mather, & Adams, 2006; Proctor, Semega, & Kollar, 2016), like environmental toxins, malnutrition, family with mental health disorders, neglect, maltreatment and abuse, violent crime, divorce and decreased stimulation. Consequently, these kids are more likely to have poor health and school failure problems. Poverty in childhood is often associated with physical and mental health problems and a higher risk for poorer academic outcomes, lower school attendance, and early school dropout. These data are dramatic, taking into account that in the USA, 4 in 10 children can be considered poor for 1 or more years and more than 1 in 10 are poor for half of their life (Ratcliffe, 2015). The situation of children growing up in poverty in developing countries is still worse. They are often not only victims of poor social conditions, but also of war, structural violence and disasters. There are millions of children living in slums all over the world, mostly in developing countries of Africa, Asia and Latin-America, but also in marginal neighbourhoods, inhabited mainly by immigrants, in UE countries and the USA. This is a complex socio-political problem, whose solution is not in the hands of Psychologists. Nevertheless, Psychology can answer some urgent questions, like for instance, searching for simple, cheap, efficient, scientifically based evaluation and intervention techniques able to help these children.

Consequently, the primary goal of the current work has been to develop Applied Behavior Analysis (ABA) diagnostic and training techniques to help children with a lack of skills, i.e., mainly social & independence skills in the case of SEN children, and mostly academic skills in the case of school failure problems. The publication of handbooks for teachers and parents with simple, cheap, efficient evaluation and training techniques for children is an essential part of this work.

## 3 Theoretical Foundations

The theoretical foundation of this work is ABA, also called Behavior Modification (Miltenberger, 2016). ABA techniques have been used for many years by numerous Psychologists to solve a broad range of psychological problems. Solving problems of persons with intellectual disability has been traditionally the main field of research and application. A great amount of information is currently available about training basic skills like instructions following, imitation, self-care and eating, as well as language and social behavior and academic skills like reading, spelling, arithmetic and using computers (Jerome, Frantino, & Sturmey, 2007). The same techniques have been applied successfully to teach the same kind of skills to children with hearing and visual impairments, with autism, or with specific learning disorders (Axe & Sainato, 2010; Green, Reid, Rollyson, & Passante, 2005; Levingston, Neef, & Cihon, 2009; Toussaint & Tiger, 2010). In the field of children with school failure problems, Adelman and Taylor (1993) analyzed different aspects of learning at school-related to academic success and failure and proposed using behavioral techniques to improve learning skills. Hallahan, Kauffman and Lloyd (1999) and Wallace, Larsen and Elksnin (1992) identified possible factors of school achievement in the individual and the family; at an individual level, they pointed to the absence of language, social and cognitive prerequisite skills as a source of failure to learn reading, writing and arithmetic. A further development has been the systematization of ABA techniques in the so-called Behavioral Skills Training (BST), that has been used successfully to teach children with autism abduction prevention skills (Johnson et al, 2005) and communication skills (Barnes, Dunning, & Rehfeldt 2011; Gianoumis, Seiverling, & Sturmey 2012). BST is a teaching package consisting of instructions, modelling, rehearsal and feedback (Ward-Horner & Sturmey, 2012). It is basically the same set of techniques used in our work to teach children with different problems: First instructions, i.e., explaining how to do a task; then modelling, i.e., demonstrating how to do the task; then rehearsal, i.e., letting the child to do the task, and finally feedback: reinforcing the correct response and correcting the incorrect response. These techniques have proved to be simple, cheap, efficient and scientific based. The current work will provide more evidence on the matter.

## 4 Settings

Being born with a deficiency is a difficult challenge for every person. The challenge is still more difficult for SEN children growing up in slums. In the next pages, I will explain the work done with children at risk in two different settings. The first one is devoted to children with intellectual disability and blindness growing up in the slums of Mexico City. In Mexico, in spite of huge governmental efforts, thousands of SEN children do not receive adequate medical and educational support. Most of them live in an affectionate familiar environment, which nevertheless does not allow them the acquisition of social, academic and independence skills, for several reasons. The most common reason is the lack of an adequate educational background by the parents. Some of these children get some medical care for some time, but no education at all. It is not rare to find blind school-age children, who never went to school. More information about this field can be found in Galindo (2009) and Galindo, Galguera, Taracena and Hinojosa (2018).

The second setting is different. The work was done in a slum-like neighbourhood not far away from Lisbon. Poverty, drugs, prostitution, police incursions and violence are common. Inhabitants are mainly immigrants from Brazil, Angola, Mozambique, Cape Verde, Ukraine and Russia. Children receive the necessary medical care and can regularly go to school, but some of them have problems at home and, consequently, at school. Some of them do not learn like other children, they repeat twice, maybe three times the first and/or the second school year, they dislike school and constantly get in trouble with schoolmates and teachers. Their problem is called school failure. In spite of impressive advances in the field, school failure remains a main educational challenge in Portugal and other European countries (Eurydice, 2011, p. 35). As usual, the problem is more frequent in poor, isolated and/or marginal strata of the population. More information about this field can be found in Galindo (2015).

## 5 Evaluation and Intervention Strategies

In general terms, the same evaluation and intervention strategies have been applied in all cases. Each child was evaluated individually, looking for the existing and failing skills, according to the expectations of family or school, taking into account the age of the kid and the everyday developmental tasks associated to that age. Learning aims were defined by Psychologists, together with the parents and/or the teachers. The core of the evaluation is always a behavioral observation of the child, but an analysis of existing medical and education reports is also included, as well as the opinions of parents and teachers. Evaluation proceeded as thick as possible, trying to identify precisely the existing and lacking skills. The diagnosis was a list of problems and failing skills for each child. On this basis, a hierarchy of intervention objectives was made, and an individually tailored behavioral training program for each skill was designed.

Each behavioral training program has roughly the same structure (see Tables 1–3): 1) a general objective, 2) skills defined in terms of specific objectives (a set of correct responses to be given by the child), 3) a definition of the previous skills necessary to learn the new skill (recurrent), 4) a pre-test (%of attained objectives/correct responses), 5) a training package based on instructions, modelling, rehearsal, and feedback, 6) a post-test (%of attained objectives/correct responses), and 7) an estimate of motivational aspects. A set of program models has been developed for each type of children, but users were encouraged to create their programs, according to the developmental needs of the child and the expectations of his/her community (family or school). Evaluation of the efficacy of the program was carried out by comparing the percentage of attained objectives before (pre-test) and after training (post-test).

In the training phase, behavioral programs were applied during at least 2 hours a week for at least one semester (15 weeks) on an individual basis (1 tutor x 1 child). Tutors were specially trained Psychology students. A token economy was introduced to motivate children (Ayllon & Azrin, 1968). The level of success of each training program was evaluated regarding a) percentage of attained objectives (or correct responses), and b) training time. A child had to attain at least 80% of objectives in a program to be considered successful. As a result of this individualised strategies, the nature of the program, the number and quality of trained skills, the duration of training and the number of trained programs greatly varied from child to child.

## 5.1 Training Children with Intellectual Disability

Participants were 4–12 years old children referred by families because of developmental problems, the absence of social and language skills. The intervention was carried out by trained tutors in training centres created in the slums of Mexico City and supported mainly by parents and relatives of the children (see Galindo et al., 2018). Every child was evaluated individually to define his/her existing or non-existing skills. On the basis of behavioral evaluations and additionally records and reports of parents, a hierarchy of problems was elaborated, taking into account the developmental needs of the child and the developmental tasks to be mastered by a child of similar age and circumstances. Then, a behavioral training program for each skill was elaborated. The following programs have been developed as a basis for further adaptation to each case: 1) Basic Behavior: Attention, Imitation, Following Instructions, Self-care (washing hands & face, brushing teeth, etc.), Motor Coordination, Discrimination of Forms & Colors, Temporal & Spatial Relationships. 2) Social and Adaptation Skills (language, playing & social norms) 3) Academic Behavior (writing, spelling, arithmetic). Attention, imitation and instruction following are considered as main basic skills that enabling the child to participate in further training

**Table 1.** Program to train attention

- Objective – The child must a) establish eye-to-eye contact with the tutor, b) look at a determined object in the room, every time he/she is requested to do so, in no more than 5 seconds.
- Definition – Attention is defined regarding the behavior of establishing visual contact with persons and objects at different distances.
- Pre-currents – The child must be able to remain sitting at least 15 minutes. Physical handicaps must be checked.
- Materials –Color cards and toys.
- Setting – Room.
- Phases – 1) pre-evaluation (pre-test), 2) training eye-to-eye contact, 3) training attention to near objects in the room, 4) training attention to objects at different distances, 5) final evaluation (post-test)

programs. Every program was designed to solve a specific problem (articulation, washing hands, writing, etc.). An example of such a program is shown in Table 1. Nevertheless, tutors were instructed to adopt a program to the specific needs and aims of the child. Behavioral Training was applied for two hours a day (10 hours x 1 week) during a semester (15 weeks). An intervention might last a few weeks or several years, depending on the children's needs. A post-test was carried out following the training.

## 5.2 Training Blind Children

Participants were 4–14 blind children referred by families because of the lack of independence and academic skills. Training was carried out by trained tutors in a training centre situated at the university campus in Mexico City (see Galindo, 2009). This centre was organized as a school for blind children, with a special curriculum divided into four intervention areas: Basic Autonomy (BA), Mobility and Orientation (M&O), Social Behavior (SB) and Academic Behavior (AB). This curriculum was created with the specific objective of preparing blind children to be integrated into the regular school. A set of behavioral training programs was applied in each area, to train specific skills. For instance, programs applied in the M&O area went from displacing alone in a closed room to travelling by bus and underground; programs in the BA area went from recognising objects through sound, smell our touch to preparing breakfast; programs in the AB area prepared the child for subject matters at school.

Every child was evaluated individually to define his/her existing or non-existing skills regarding the existing programs, in the same way already explained. By the hierarchy of non-existing skills, behavioral training programs were elaborated and applied. An example of such a program is shown in Table 2. As usual, tutors were

**Table 2.** Program to train displacement with a cane

| | |
|---|---|
| General objective: The child must be able to walk, at least 1½ km, in less than 1 hour, in different streets of his/her neighbourhood, using the cane. Pre-currents: Programs of BA level I, M&O level 1 and SB level 1, and social norms. | |
| **Specific objectives** | **Steps** |
| To hold the cane according to rules a, b, c | a), b), c) |
| To walk 20 meters in 7minutes on an even floor. | a), b), c) |
| To walk 50 meters with obstacles. | a), b) |
| To displace downstairs and upstairs. | a), b), c) |
| To walk along the street with the cane, using the walls as a point of reference. | a), b), c) |
| To cross five different streets, with help. | a), b), c) |
| To displace from the training centre to bus stop, using the cane, without help. | a), b), c) |

instructed to adopt every program to the specific needs and aims of the child. Behavioral training was applied for two hours a day (10 hours x 1 week) during a semester (15 weeks). A child was considered ready for school when he had attained successfully all skills defined by the curriculum. A post-test was carried out following the training.

## 5.3 Training Children with Problems of School Failure

Participants were 6–12 school children referred by teachers because of problems of school failure. The intervention was carried on in a primary school (ISCED 1) situated in a slum-like neighbourhood in Lisbon (see Galindo, 2015). School success was defined regarding a set of skills proposed by teachers. School failure was then understood as a lack of one or more of these skills. Consequently, the specific objectives of these interventions are 1) to develop intervention techniques based on school defined skills for ISCED 1, 2) to apply systematically training programs to attain those skills, and 3) to publish a handbook containing the techniques.

Before the intervention, the existing and non existing skills, as well as the possible aims of the training were defined together with the teacher. All information was used to elaborate a hierarchy of problems. On this basis, an intervention strategy was designed, elaborating specific training programs for the child. The following programs have been developed as a basis for further adaptation to each case: 1) Basic behavior (pre-currents): Self-care, motor coordination, discrimination of forms & colors, pre-reading, pre-writing, verbal behavior, temporal and spatial relationships, 2) Academic behavior (first, second, and third school years): Reading,

Table 3. Program to recognise letters

General objective: The child must be able to recognise all letters of the Portuguese alphabet.
Specific objectives: The child must be able to identify and reproduce the sound of all alphabet letters, 1) handwritten, lowercase letter, 2) handwritten, capital letters, 3) print, lower case letters and print, capital letters
Definition: A response is correct if the child a) identifies a letter presented by the tutor, and 2) reproduces the sound of a letter presented by the tutor.
Pre-currents: Basic repertoires and language without articulation problems.
Materials: Cards with letters (see table 3)
Place: A working room or classroom
Procedure:
1) Pre-test: All letters are presented.
2) Training: A package of instructions, modelling, rehearsal, and feedback.
   a) Handwritten, lower case letters.
   b) Handwritten, capital letters.
   c) Print, lower case letters.
   d) Print, capital letters.
   The child must be able to respond correctly, without help, to the same question in five successive trials.
3) Post-test: All letters are presented.
Training has been successful if the child attains at least 80% of correct responses.

Writing, Environment, Mathematics, and Portuguese, and 3) Social behavior. Every program was designed to solve a specific problem (writing, spelling, articulation, etc.). An example of such a program is shown in table 3. Behavioral Training was applied for two hours a week (2 sessions x 1 hour) during a semester (15 weeks). The intervention was carried on by tutors in different rooms at school. An intervention might last a few weeks or the whole semester, depending on the children's needs. A post-test was carried out following the training.

# 6 Results

Hundreds of children with problems of intellectual disability, blindness, deafness, physical deficiencies, language disorders, ADHD, specific learning disorders, and autism have been taught in the training centres of Mexico City (see Galindo et al., 2018), as well children with problems of school failure in Portugal (see Galindo, 2015).

**Table 4.** Case 1 of male, eight years old with intellectual disability. Trained skills and obtained results in evaluations before and after training; one session = two hours.

| Skill | 1st Test | Training | 2nd Test |
|---|---|---|---|
| Sitting 30 minutes | 33 | 12 sessions | 100 |
| Attention | 100 | ---- | |
| Following Instructions | 25 | 33 sessions | 90–100 |
| Imitation | 20 | No | |
| Motor coordination | 80 | ---- | |
| Verbal imitation | 0 | No | |
| Recognition objects | 0 | No | |
| Answer questions | 0 | No | |

Some illustrative cases of these children will be presented in the following pages, to give a better picture of the procedures and techniques used during evaluation and training.

Case 1 (see Table 4) is an 8-years-old boy with an intellectual disability. The family lived in very poor conditions, and the child had never received any special medical care nor education. Parents informed he was "hyperactive", dependent and did not show any self- care skills, but some disruptive behaviors, like tantrums. Behavioral observations, devoted mainly to basic skills, showed he had attention (100%) but deficiencies in instructions following (25%), and imitation (20%). His motor coordination was good enough (80%), but he had huge language problems: Verbal imitation (0%), recognition of objects (0%), and answering questions (0%). Concerning hyperactivity, sitting quietly in a chair for 30 minutes was defined as a good behavioral objective. A first evaluation showed he was able to sit only 10 minutes (33%). A hierarchy of problems was defined. The first objective was to attain was "sitting quietly for 30 minutes"; it was attained in 12 one-hour sessions. The next step was training skills for following instructions; the child learned to follow 90–100% of given instructions in 33 one-hour sessions. This child illustrates the strategy applied to train difficult cases: The first step is always training attention, imitation and following instructions. Here, a previous step was necessary, namely, to get the child in a chair for 30 minutes. The next step should be the training of imitation and language skills.

Case 2 (see Table 5) is a 7-years-old boy with an intellectual disability. He had received no education, but some psychiatric attention. According to the family, treatment showed no results and controlling the child was increasing difficult. Behavioral observations showed he had low attention (65%) but no deficiencies in instructions following (100%) nor imitation (100%). His motor coordination was good enough (95%), but he had language problems. Further evaluation of language and social behavior showed verbal imitation was good (100%), and functional

Table 5. Case 2 of male, seven years old with intellectual disability. Trained skills and obtained results in evaluations before and after training; one session = two hours.

| Area | Program | 1st Evaluation (%Attained Objectives) | 2nd Evaluation (%Attained Objectives) |
|---|---|---|---|
| **Basic autonomy** | Tactile discrimination | 56.7 | 100 |
| | Washing hands/face | 65 | 100 |
| | Brushing teeth | 68 | 100 |
| | Put on shoes | 45 | 100 |
| | Cleaning shoes | 0 | 100 |
| **Socialisation** | No data | | |
| **Mobility & orientation** | Space-temporal skills | 25 | 100 |
| | Recognising objects | 14.5 | 100 |
| | Displace no guide | 0 | 100 |
| | Displacement guide | 0 | 100 |
| | Displacement cane | 0 | 100 |
| | Bus & subway | 0 | 100 |
| | Community services | 0 | 100 |
| **Academic Behavior** | 15 School subjects | 100 | 100 |
| | | 33 | 33 |
| | | 0 | 0 |
| | | 0 | 0 |
| | | 0 | 0 |
| | | 100 | 100 |
| | | 0 | 100 |
| | | 0 | 100 |
| | | 0 | 100 |
| | | 0 | 100 |
| | | 0 | 0 |
| | | 100 | 100 |
| | | 33 | 33 |
| | | 100 | 100 |
| | | 0 | 0 |

language was a relative good established, but there were clear deficiencies in the articulation of /s/ (40%) and /r/ (0%). On the other hand, he was constantly out of his chair. It was decided to solve articulation problems and apply for a training program in recognising forms (0%), to start the establishment of cognitive pre-academic skills. At the same time, a program to train "sitting in his chair for 30 minutes" was applied. Table 5 shows the child could attain 100% of attention skills in 5 one-hour sessions. Articulation problems of /s/ was reasonably solved (86%) in 11 one-hour-sessions and a good advance was obtained in the articulation of /r/ (45%) in 7 sessions. Additionally, the child learned recognising forms (100%) in 35 sessions. This child illustrates the strategy applied in a persistent case, namely children with middle difficulties, concentrated mainly in language and social interaction.

Case 3 (see table 6) is a blind 8-years-old girl, who lost her vision in the early infancy due to a disease. The family gave the child an affectionate environment and good medical care, but no schooling, due to financial problems. The girl showed a relatively good social, emotional & cognitive development, but social isolation and no independence nor self-care skills. Training in the above-described centre for blind children proceeded during two years. The first year was devoted to an intensive socialisation training (no quantitative data are available). An evaluation made at the beginning of the second year (table 6, first evaluation) showed the following deficiencies:

a) Basic Autonomy: tactile discrimination (56.7%), washing hands and face (65%), brushing teeth (68%), put on shoes (45%), cleaning shoes (0%).
b) Mobility and Orientation: space-temporal relations (25%), recognizing objects (14.5%), displacement without a guide (0%), displacement with guide (0%), displacement with cane (0%), displacement with bus and subway (0%), using community services (0%).
c) Academic Behavior, i.e., school subjects of ICED 1 (reading, spelling, natural sciences, mathematics): Four items with 100%, two items with 33 %, nine items with 0%.

The child was trained one year, 10 hours a week, first in Basic Autonomy, secondly in M&O and then in Academic Behavior. Table 6 shows the results. The child advanced to 100% in all programs of Basic Autonomy and M&O. She attained 100% skills in some school subjects but remained by 0% in others (mainly mathematics) and by 33% in one. The child had learned a great amount of independence, but she was not still prepared to attend the regular school. Additionally, tutors observed the girl was still shy and nervous in some social situations. Consequently, it was decided to go on with training one more semester.

Case 4 (see table 7) is a 10-years-old girl attending the second school year, referred by the teacher because of academic and behavior problems. The girl showed a relatively good social, emotional & cognitive development, but clear signs of physical neglect, like dirty clothes and unwashed hands, face and hair. The mother lived from prostitution and used to send the girl to school with an

Table 6. Case 3 of female, eight years old. Training programs and obtained results in evaluations before and after training.

| Area | Program | 1st Evaluation (%attained objectives) | 2nd Evaluation (%attained objectives) |
|---|---|---|---|
| **Basic autonomy** | Tactile discrimination | 56.7 | 100 |
| | Washing hands/face | 65 | 100 |
| | Brushing teeth | 68 | 100 |
| | Put on shoes | 45 | 100 |
| | Cleaning shoes | 0 | 100 |
| **Socialisation** | No data | | |
| **Mobility & orientation** | Space-temporal skills | 25 | 100 |
| | Recognising objects | 14.5 | 100 |
| | Displace no guide | 0 | 100 |
| | Displacement guide | 0 | 100 |
| | Displacement cane | 0 | 100 |
| | Bus & subway | 0 | 100 |
| | Community services | 0 | 100 |
| **Academic Behavior** | 15 School subjects | 100 | 100 |
| | | 33 | 33 |
| | | 0 | 0 |
| | | 0 | 0 |
| | | 0 | 0 |
| | | 100 | 100 |
| | | 0 | 100 |
| | | 0 | 100 |
| | | 0 | 100 |
| | | 0 | 100 |
| | | 0 | 0 |
| | | 100 | 100 |
| | | 33 | 33 |
| | | 100 | 100 |
| | | 0 | 0 |

**Table 7.** Case 4 of female, ten years old, 2nd year of school. Training programs and obtained results in evaluations before and after training.

| Program | Pre-test (January) | Post-test (July) |
| --- | --- | --- |
| Self-care | 70% | 85% |
| Forms discrimination | 50% | 100% |
| Verbal comprehension | 40% | 100% |
| Spatial-temporal skills | 70% | 100% |

older brother. According to the teacher, she had repeated three times the first school year; she had no interest in academic activities, she was aggressive and was avoided by schoolmates. Behavioral observations showed she had deficiencies in reading, spelling and mathematics. A more precise evaluation showed a lack of pre-academic skills: Discrimination of forms (50%), verbal comprehension (40%) and spatial-temporal relationships (70%). A hierarchy of problems was made, with self-care skills on the top, and then pre-academic skills. She was trained during one semester, 4 hours a week. Table 7 shows the results. The girl advanced from 70% to 85% of self-care skills and attained 100% of objectives in discrimination of forms, verbal comprehension and spatial-temporal relationships. According to the teacher, after training the child showed much better social behavior, but only small improvements were evident in academic behavior. This case illustrates the evaluation and intervention strategies applied to children with problems of school failure, and also a common situation: Unfortunately, the advances of a child are not always immediately evident for the teacher. For instance, training social and pre-academic skills has no immediate consequences on academic behavior.

## 7 Conclusion

Results show an improvement of trained behavior in all cases, as a consequence of intervention. Similar results have been reported by authors, applying ABA techniques in training and rehabilitation of SEN children (Axe & Sainato, 2010; Barnes, et al., 2011; Gianoumis et al., 2012; Green et al., 2005; Jerome et al., 2007; Levingston et al., 2009; Toussaint & Tiger, 2010) or children with school failure problems (Adelman & Taylor, 1993; Hallahan et al., 1999; and Wallace et al., 1992). Parent and teachers reported significant positive changes in all cases. However, parent and teachers sometimes complained a child behaved better, although he still had problems. This is assumed because rehabilitation is a process for the whole life. Training independence skills open new development possibilities to a child, and consequently creates new training challenges: now it is necessary to learn skills to master school tasks. Nevertheless, these results seem to show applied programs are successful in training a set of skills, whose absence may cause further development problems. Probably, the most important result of this work has been the publication of handbooks for psychologists, teachers and parents, containing evaluation & intervention techniques for SEN children and children with school failures problems (Galindo, 2009; 2015; Galindo et al., 2018). Notwithstanding, more research is needed with other children, skills, ages, settings, etc., to contribute to the solution of the problems of SEN children and children with school failure at an individual level.

## 8 Affiliation

Prof. Dr. Edgar Galindo
Institution: Universidade de Evora (University of Evora)
Address: Departamento de Psicologia, 7005-345 Evora, Portugal
E-mail: edgar_galindo@hotmail.com

## 9 References

Adelman, H. S., & Taylor, L. (1993). *Learning problems and learning disabilities: Moving forward.* Pacific Grove, CA: Brooks/Cole Publishing Company.

Axe, J.B., & Sainato, D.M. (2010). Matrix training of preliteracy skills with preschoolers with autism. *Journal of Applied Behavior Analysis, 43,* 635–652. doi: 10.1901/jaba.2010.43-635

Ayllon, T., & Azrin, N.H. (1968). *The Token Economy: A Motivational System for Therapy and Rehabilitation.* Prentice Hall: Englewood Cliffs.

Baltes, P. B., Staudinger, U. M., & Lindenberger, U. (1999). Lifespan psychology: Theory and application to intellectual functioning. *Annual Review of Psychology, 50,* 471–507.

Barnes, C. S., Dunning, J. L., & Rehfeldt, R. A. (2011). An evaluation of strategies for training staff to implement the picture exchange communication system. *Research in Autism Spectrum Disorders, 5,* 1574–1583. doi: 10.1015/jrsad.2011.03.003

Bijou, S. W. (1963). Theory and research in mental (developmental) retardation. *The Psychological Record, 13,* 95–110.

Bronfenbrenner, U. (2004). *Making Human Beings Human: Bioecological Perspectives on Human Development.* Newbury Park, California: Sage Publications.

Catalano, R. F., Loeber, R., & and McKinney, K. C. (1999). School and Community Interventions to Prevent Serious and Violent Offending. *Juvenile, Justice Bulletin.* Retrieved on June 8, 2017 from http://www.ncjrs.gov/pdffiles1/ojjdp/177624.pdf

Darensbourg, A. M., & Blake, J. J. (2013). Predictors of achievement in African American students at risk for academic failure: The roles of achievement values and behavioral engagement. *Psychology in the Schools, 50*(10), 1044–1059, doi: 10.1002/pits.21730

Eurydice. (2011). *Grade Retention during Compulsory Education in Europe: Regulations and Statistics*. Brussels: Eurydice.

Frederickson, N., & Cline, T. (2015). *Special education needs, inclusion and diversity* (3rd edition). New York: McGraw Hills.

Galindo, E. (2015). *Tratamento do insucesso escolar com técnicas da psicología: Manual prático* [Treatment of school failure with techniques of Psychology: A practical handbook]. Lisboa: Livros Horizonte.

Galindo, E. (Ed.). (2009) *Psicología y educación especial* [Psychology and special education] (2nd. Ed.). Mexico: Ed. Trillas.

Galindo, E., Galguera, M.I., Taracena, E., & Hinojosa, G. (2018). *La modificación de conducta en la educación especial. Diagnóstico y programas* [Behavior modification in special education: Diagnosis and programs] (5th edition). Mexico: Editorial Trillas.

Gianoumis, S., Seiverling, L., & Sturmey, P. (2012). The effects of behavior skills training on correct teacher implementation of natural language paradigm teaching skills and child behavior. *Behavioral Interventions, 27*(2), 57–74. doi: 10.1002/bin.1334

Green, C. W., Reid, D. H., Rollyson, J. H., & Passante, S. C. (2005). An enriched teaching program for reducing resistance and indices of unhappiness among individuals with profound multiple disabilities. *Journal of Applied Behavior Analysis, 38*, 221–233. doi: 10.1901/jaba.2005.4-04

Hallahan, D., Kauffman, J., & Lloyd, J. W. (1999). *Introduction to learning disabilities*. Boston: Allyn & Bacon.

Hamre, B. K., & Pianta, R. C. (2005). Can instructional and emotional support in the first-grade classroom make a difference for children at risk of school failure? *Child development, 76*(5), 949–967. doi: 10.1111/j.1467-8624.2005.00889.x

Heward, W. L. (2017). *Exceptional children: An introduction to special education* (11$^{TH}$ edition). Upper Saddle River, Nova Jersey: Pearson Prentice Hall.

Huffman, L. C., Mehlinger, S. L., & Kerivan, A. S. (2000). *Risk factors for academic and behavioral problems at the beginning of school*. Stanford: The Child and Mental Health Foundation Agencies Network.

Jerome, J., Frantino, E. P., & Sturmey, P. (2007). The effects of errorless learning and backward chaining on the acquisition of internet skills in adults with developmental disabilities. *Journal of Applied Behavior Analysis, 40*, 185–189. doi: 10.1901/jaba.2007.41-06

Knudsen, E. I. (2004). Sensitive periods in the development of the brain and behavior. *Journal of Cognitive Neuroscience, 16*(8), 1412–1425. doi: 10.1162/0898929042304796

Levingston, H. B., Neef, N. A., & Cihon, T. M. (2009). The effects of teaching precurrent behaviors on children's solution of multiplication and division word problems. *Journal of Applied Behavior Analysis*, 42, 361-367. doi: 10.1901/jaba.2009.42-361

Martin, E., Del Barrio, C., Montero, I., Fernandez, I., Gutierrez, H., & Ochaita, E. (2003). La violencia en la escuela (Violence at school). In A. Marchesi, & C. Hernandez Gil (Eds.). *El fracaso escolar. Una perspectiva internacional* [School failure. An international perspective] (pp. 129-148). Madrid: Alianza Editorial.

Mash, E. J., & Wolfe, D. (2016). *Abnormal child Psychology* (6th edition). Belmont CA: Wadsworth Publishing Co.

Mather, M., & Adams, D. (2006). *A KIDS COUNT/PRB report on Census 2000: The risk of negative child outcomes in low-income families.* KIDS COUNT and Population Reference Bureau. Retrieved on August 14, 2017 from http://www.aecf.org/upload/PublicationFiles/ DA3622H1234.pdf

McClelland, M. M., Morrison, F. J., & Holmes, D. L. (2000). Children at risk for early academic problems: The role of learning-related social skills. *Early Childhood Research Quarterly*, 15(3), 307-329. Retrieved from https://doi.org/10.1016/S0885-2006(00)00069-7

Mendoza, M. G. (2012). *Crisis y educación en el México actual* [Crisis and education in present Mexico]. Toluca: Universidad Pedagógica Nacional.

Miltenberger, R.G. (2016). *Behavior modification. Principles and procedures* (6th edition). Boston: Cengage Learning.

Organization for Economic Co-operation and Development [OECD] (1998). *Overcoming failure at school.* Paris: OECD.

Proctor, B., Semega, J., & Kollar, M. (2016). Income and poverty in the United States: 2015. *Current Population Reports.* Retrieved on August 15, 2017 from http://www.census.gov/content/dam/Census/library/publications/2016/demo/p60-256.pdf

Ratcliffe, C. (2015). *Child poverty and adult success.* Urban Institute. Retrieved on July 2, 2017 from http://www.urban.org/sites/default/files/alfresco/publication-pdfs/2000369-Child-Poverty-and-Adult-Success.pdf

Rieber, R. W., & Carton, A. S. (Ed.) (1993). *The Collected Works of L. S. Vygotsky. Vol. 2: The Fundamentals of Defectology.* New York: Plenum Publishing Corporation.

Sapp, M. (1996). Irrational beliefs that can lead to academic failure for African American middle school students who are academically at-risk. *Journal of Rational-Emotive and Cognitive-Behavior Therapy*, 14(2), 123-134.

Toussaint K. A., & Tiger J. H. (2010). Teaching early braille literacy skills within a stimulus equivalence paradigm to children with degenerative visual impairments. *Journal of Applied Behavior Analysis*, 43, 181-194. doi: 10.1901/jaba.2010.43-181

Wallace, G., Larsen, S., & Elksnin, L. (1992). *Educational Assessment of Learning Problems*. Boston: Allyn & Bacon.

Ward-Horner, J. and Sturmey P. (2012). Component analysis of behavior skills training in functional analysis. *Behavioral Interventions, 27*(2), 75–92. doi: 10.1002/bin.1339

Whitman, T. L., & Johnston, M. (1983). Teaching addition and subtraction to educable mentally retarded children: A group self-instructional approach. *Behavior Therapy, 14*, 127–143.

Wood, D. K., Frank, A. R., & Wacker, D. P. (1998). Teaching multiplication facts to students with learning disabilities. *Journal of Applied Behavior Analysis, 31*(3), 323–338. doi: 10.1901/jaba.1998.31-323

Dian Sari Utami & Evelin Witruk

# Parenting Stressors and Positive Coping among Indonesian Parents with a Deaf or Hard-of-Hearing Schoolchild

**Abstract:** Hearing parents reported some problems while parenting their deaf or hard-of-hearing schoolchildren, such as parenting stress. This paper aims to understand the source of stress and parental coping strategy during parenting a deaf or hard-of-hearing schoolchild for Indonesian parents. Data was collected using qualitative approach by distributing open questionnaires in four special schools in Yogyakarta, Indonesia. There were 40 parents with deaf or hard-of-hearing schoolchildren at grade 4 to 6. Method of data analysis was conducted using content analysis. The findings show that the source of stress when parenting the deaf or hard-of-hearing schoolchildren are coming from parents itself, children, and media. Further, it is found that parents use some coping strategies, such as self-regulation, active communication, seeking help, giving educational concern, become permissive, and applying the spiritual approach to their deaf or hard-of-hearing children. The implication of this study is focusing on the positive parenting program for families with deaf or hard-of-hearing schoolchildren. Later on, it is suggested for future investigation to explore the family resources, such as parenting values and psychological aspects, which will strengthen the positive parenting within families with deaf or hard-of-hearing schoolchildren.

**Keywords:** parenting stress, positive coping, deaf or hard-of-hearing schoolchildren, Indonesian parents

## 1 Introduction

Having a deaf or hard-of-hearing (D/HH) child is a challenge for parents, particularly for hearing parents. Hearing parents report stressful condition while parenting their D/HH child. In Indonesia, D/HH schoolchildren grade 4th to 6th are in a transition phase of academic life from primary to secondary school. This condition gives more stress for the D/HH children itself and their hearing parents. Despite of the communication problems or misunderstanding that occur in most hearing parents due to D/HH condition of the child, others problems might also become the source of the stressful condition among parents with a D/HH child. Also, as mentioned in some studies, the stressful condition faced by parents is related to communication problems, educational concerns, financial problems, behavior problems, future safety and security of the schoolchildren with D/HH (Hintermair, 2006; Pipp-Siegel, Sedey, & Yoshinaga-Itano, 2002; Quittner, Barker, Cruz, Snell, Grimley, Botteri, & the CDaCI Investigative Team, 2010).

Further, in a previous study through an interview and observation, some Indonesian parents reported some challenges raising the D/HH child, such as stigmatization from neighbourhood and child's emotional problems at home (Santoso, Yuliani, Utami, Salim, & Sugiyanto, 2003). Some families with D/HH children also reported of parental divorce due to the difficulties raising the child and this became problems between parents to blame each other.

Most studies focused on the parenting stress with D/HH in early childhood (Lederberg & Golbach, 2002; Pipp-Siegel et al., 2002; Quittner et al., 2010) and less study engaged with the parenting stress of children with D/HH during adolescence. Thus, it is necessary to understand the parenting issues of raising D/HH children during adolescence (Zaidman-Zait, 2014). Particularly, the study of parenting children with D/HH during school transition from primary to secondary schools (i.e., 4th to 6th Grade) has not been found in the previous research.

Thus, the author considered to make a follow-up through this study. It is aimed to understand the source of parenting stress and the positive coping strategy used by Indonesian hearing parents with a school-age D/HH child.

# 2 Theoretical Review

## 2.1 Deaf or Hard-of-Hearing Schoolchildren

World Health Organization (WHO, 2017) defines deaf or hearing loss as "a person who is not able to hear as well as someone with normal hearing – hearing thresholds of 25 dB or better in both ears". Whereas 'hard-of-hearing' defines further by WHO (2017) as difficulties to hear a sound and communicate spoken the language from hearing aids, cochlear implants, and other devices.

In the developmental lifespan, D/HH schoolchildren have different stages compared with hearing children at the same age. D/HH children share developmental experiences that are less than average. Further, problems related to the developmental stage among D/HH children and adults are communicative deprivation, difficulties in their families of origin, less than adequate educational experiences, and continuing stigma and prejudice (Greenberg & Kusché, 1998).

Schneider (2001) mentions in one study that D/HH children face difficulties during their life stages, such as identity problems, exhausting, lower life happiness and social competence, and less trust. Therefore, it is crucial to present knowledge for hearing parents with D/HH children regarding parenting to enhance positive parent-child relationships with D/HH children.

Nevertheless, intellectual ability among D/HH children seems no differ with hearing children regarding IQ (Prinz, Strong, Kuntze, Friedman, Moyers, & Helman, 1996). Even so, interestingly, evidence shows that the left hemisphere of the brain is also the primary site responsible for sign language among D/HH children (Emmorey, 2002).

Furthermore, a supportive home environment shows evidence to influence D/HH children having a higher-achievement at schools. This is due to the involvement of families in the child's education, parents seek knowledge about the child's condition to provide guidance, parents have high expectations for achievement, do not try to overprotect their child, and participate along with their D/HH child in the Deaf community are motivating the child to be successful and perform achievement (Schirmer, 2001).

In Indonesia, D/HH children are provided facilities for education, such as special schools for children who affected with auditory problems. There are also inclusive schools which provide the same chance for all children to learn together. Nevertheless, many parents feel confidence to bring their D/HH child to the special schools to get a proper education in accordance with the child's ability despite of their deaf or hard-of-hearing condition.

## 2.2 Parenting Deaf or Hard-of-Hearing Children, Stress, and Coping Strategy

The parenting stress on raising the D/HH children strive the family to maintain the balance of the changing situation and the demands of the family and the community. The change itself is stressful for an organism; however, a stressor is anything that potentially leads the individual to change (Boss, 2002). Some stressors are neutral and lead to a state of stress when they are required to change (Boss, 2002). The condition in a state of stress will force hearing parents cope, adjust, and adapt to the changing situation in the family due to the D/HH of the child. This stress condition of the hearing parents will influence the behavior problems of children with D/HH and often more complicated by the language delays due to the reduced of hearing (Quittner et al., 2010). Many researchers related with parental issues of children with D/HH have discussed mostly about parenting stress using quantitative approach (Lederberg & Golbach, 2002; Plotkin, Brice, & Reesman, 2014; Sarant & Garrard, 2014; Zaidman-Zait, Most, Tarrasch, Haddad-eid, & Brand, 2016) than explored it using qualitative approach about parenting problems and coping strategies among fathers and mothers with a D/HH child.

In comparison with the issues of parenting stress and problems of children with D/HH in many previous studies, it is relatively little known about the positive perspective of hearing parents with a D/HH schoolchild. One study using a qualitative approach in the application of positive psychology among parents with D/HH children between one to fourteen years of age has shown the positive perceptions of parents during raising their D/HH children (Szarkowski & Brice, 2016). It has been mentioned that parents reported as knowing the child, appreciating everyday positives, increasing involvement with the child, relishing the highs, taking less for granted, letting go, learning, advocating, and experiencing personal growth. Another study shows the pathways model of perceived social support, family well-being, quality of parenting, and child resilience will emphasize strength, health, competence and family empowerment (Armstrong, Birnie-Lefcovitch, & Ungar, 2005).

## 3 Method

### 3.1 Sample

This study applied a qualitative research method using a nonprobability sampling (i.e., purposive sampling method). Later, the sample in this qualitative study is called "participants". The characteristics of participants in this study were hearing parents in Indonesia with a deaf or a hard-of-hearing schoolchild from grade 4th to 6th, without any disabilities and chronic illness. There were 40 hearing parents (21 mothers; 19 fathers) aged between 31 to 35 years (32.5%), 36 to 40 years (22.5%), 41 to 45 years (17.5%), and above 45 years (27.5%). Parents were recruited from four special schools in Yogyakarta region, Indonesia.

### 3.2 Measurement Tools

The data collection was administered using open questionnaires for hearing parents with D/HH schoolchildren. The questions were as followed:

a) *"I love my child very much. Nevertheless, sometimes I have problems while parenting them."* Which problems you faced while parenting your child?
b) *"I try to solve my parenting problems. Some strategies I use are…"*

Parents were asked their willingness to volunteer in this study through signing an informed consent and understood the procedure and the ethical consideration.

## 4 Results

Concerning the texts related to parenting issues from the perspectives of parents with D/HH schoolchild, three groupings of themes are found as results. The source of stress when parenting the deaf or hard-of-hearing schoolchildren are coming from parents itself, children, and media.

Further, it is found that parents use some affirmative coping strategies, such as self-regulation, active communication, seeking help, giving educational concern, and applying the spiritual approach to their deaf or hard-of-hearing children (see Table 1).

Most of the Indonesian hearing parents in this study used active communication to deal with the adversity of language of their D/HH schoolchildren. Seeking support from friends, families, and others are the relevant keys to buffer with the stressful situation while parenting their D/HH schoolchildren. Hearing parents will attempt to regulate their selves through being patient in the uncertainty adversity situation when raising their D/HH schoolchildren.

## 5 Conclusion

The urgent stressor faced by Indonesian parents with a D/HH schoolchild is language misunderstanding due to the child's condition. Thus, it is crucial for hearing parents develop their meanings of communication with their D/HH

Table 1. Results of content analysis about parenting D/HH schoolchildren

| Themes | Category | Subcategory | Phrase frequency |
| --- | --- | --- | --- |
| Source of stress | Parents | Less time with the child | 2 |
| | | Lack of emotional control | 3 |
| | Children | Indiscipline | 8 |
| | | Lack of self-confidence | 3 |
| | | Language misunderstanding | 20 |
| | Environment | Media | 4 |
| | | Peers | 4 |
| | | School's facilitate | 4 |
| Coping strategy | Self-regulation | Be grateful | 8 |
| | | Acceptance | 8 |
| | | Be patient | 10 |
| | | Positive thinking | 6 |
| | | Giving love | 3 |
| | Active communication | Frequent, open, repeated, persuasive, appreciate, give advice, talk heart to heart | 20 |
| | | Sign language | 4 |
| | Seeking help | Family, friends, other support | 12 |
| | Giving educational concern | Formal learning | 5 |
| | Spiritual approach | Guidance in life | 3 |
| | | Religious activity | 5 |

schoolchild and provide more visual and interactive way to transmit the messages or the information. It is suggested that parents can communicate with their D/HH children using sign-language communication early and consistently or applying consistent communication ways with the D/HH schoolchildren. As a result, their D/HH children can develop verbal, numerical, and spatial reasoning first and consistent spoken-language connection with their hearing children peer (Bandurski & Galkowski, 2004).

Coping study that found in this study showed that Indonesian hearing parents applied affirmative ways to face the stressors while parenting the D/HH schoolchildren. This is also relevant with the previous study from Utami (2018) that Indonesian parents use positive cognitive-emotion regulation, such as acceptance, positive reappraisal, and positive refocusing. The usage of acceptance and positive refocusing are helping the individual to experience their selves to what has happened (Potthoff, Garnefski, Miklósi, Ubbiali, Domínguez-Sánchez, Martins, Witthöft, & Kraaij, 2016) and to think other pleasant matters instead of the actual event (Garnefski, Kraaij, & Spinhoven, 2001) to maintain harmony within society.

Further, the understanding of parental issues in parenting the children with D/HH, such as problems, strategies, and outcomes of the parenting process, will give practice benefit for hearing parents as lesson learned to know how raising the D/HH children in the school grade forth to sixth and how to cope with some parenting problems.

Some limitations of this study are also evaluated. Number of participants and a survey method using open questionnaires, however, could not capture the effectiveness of stressors and affirmative coping strategies used by the hearing parents and its impacts. Nevertheless, results in this study could give some recommendations for future research as well. It is suggested that in-depth interview among hearing parents and observation in a natural setting (i.e., at home) should be applied for further study to understand the parent-child relationships between hearing parents and their D/HH schoolchildren. Observations at special schools, particularly among the hearing parents during the class activity and teaching break-time become an idea to see the consistency on parenting D/HH schoolchildren and its impacts on D/HH schoolchildren development (i.e., emotional and behavior).

# 6 Affiliations

Dr. Dian Sari Utami
Institution: Department of Psychology, Islamic University of Indonesia
Address: Kampus Terpadu Universitas Islam Indonesia, Jurusan Psikologi, Jalan Kaliurang Km 14.5, Sleman 55584, Yogyakarta, Indonesia
E-mail: dian.utami@uii.ac.id

Prof. Dr. Evelin Witruk
Institution: Institute of Psychology, University of Leipzig
Address: Staedtiches Kaufhaus, Neumarkt 9-19, 04109 Leipzig, Germany
E-mail: witruk@uni-leipzig.de

# 7 References

Armstrong, M. I., Birnie-Lefcovitch, S., & Ungar, M. T. (2005). Pathways between social support, family well-being, quality of parenting, and child resilience: What we know. *Journal of Child and Family Studies, 14*(2), 269–281.

Bandurski, M., & Galkowski, T. (2004). The development of analogical reasoning in deaf children and their parents' communication mode. *Journal of Deaf Studies and Deaf Education, 9*(2), 153–175.

Boss, P. (2002). *Family stress: A contextual approach.* Thousand Oaks, CA: Sage.

Emmorey, K. (2002). *Language, cognition, and the brain: Insights from sign language research*. Mahwah, NJ: Lawrence Erlbaum.

Garnefski, N., Kraaij, V., & Spinhoven, P. (2001). *CERQ: Manual for the use of the Cognitive Emotion Regulation Questionnaire. A questionnaire measuring cognitive coping strategies*. Leiderdorp: DATEC.

Greenberg, M. T., & Kusché, C. (1998). Preventive intervention for school-age deaf children: The PATHS curriculum. *Journal of Deaf Studies and Deaf Education, 3*, 49–63.

Hintermair, M. (2006). Parental resources, parental stress, and socio-emotional development of deaf and hard-of-hearing children. *Journal of Deaf Studies and Deaf Education, 11*(4), 493–513.

Lederberg, A. R., & Golbach, T. (2002). Parenting stress and social support in hearing mothers of deaf and hearing children: A longitudinal study. *Journal of Deaf Studies and Deaf Education, 7*(4), 330–345.

Pipp-Siegel, S., Sedey, A. L., & Yoshinaga-Itano, C. (2002). Predictors of parental stress in mothers of young children with hearing loss. *Journal of Deaf Studies and Deaf Education, 7*, 1–17.

Plotkin, R. M., Brice, P. J., & Reesman, J. H. (2014). It is not just stress: Parent personality in raising a deaf child. *Journal of Deaf Studies and Deaf Education, 19*(3), 347–357.

Potthoff, S., Garnefski, N., Miklósi, M., Ubbiali, A., Domínguez-Sánchez, F. J., Martins, E. C., Witthöft, M., & Kraaij, V. (2016). Cognitive emotion regulation and psychopathology across cultures: A comparison between six European countries. *Personality and Individual Differences, 98*, 218–224.

Prinz, P. M., Strong, M., Kuntze, M., Vincent, J., Friedman, J., Moyers, P. P., & Helman, E. (1996). A path to literacy through ASL and English for Deaf children. In C. E. Johnson & J. H. V. Gibert (Eds.), *Children's language* (Vol. 9, pp. 235–251). Mahwah, NJ: Lawrence Erlbaum.

Quittner, A. L., Barker, D. H., Cruz, I., Snell, C., Grimley, M. E., Botteri, M., & the CDaCI Investigative Team. (2010). Parenting stress among parents of deaf and hearing children: Associations with language delays and behavior problems. *Parenting, Science and Practice, 10*, 136–155.

Santoso, A. B., Yuliani, G., Utami, D. S., Salim, D., & Sugiyanto. (2003). *Terapi Musik untuk meningkatkan emotional well-being pada anak tunarungu* [Music therapy to increase emotional well-being among hearing impaired children] (LKIP-DIKTI Research Report). Yogyakarta: Fakultas Psikologi Universitas Gadjah Mada.

Sarant, J., & Garrard, P. (2014). Parenting stress in parents of children with Cochlear Implants: Relationships among parent stress, child language, and unilateral versus bilateral implants. *Journal of Deaf Studies and Deaf Education, 19*(1), 85–106.

Schirmer, B. R. (2001). *Psychological, social, and educational dimensions of deafness.* Needham Heights, MA: Allyn & Bacon.

Schneider, S. (2001). *Hörgeschädigte Kindern: Ratgeber für Eltern* [Hearing impaired children: Advice for parents]. Ratingen: Oberstebrink Verlag.

Szarkowski, A., & Brice, P. J. (2016). Hearing parents' appraisals of parenting a deaf or hard-of-hearing child: Application of a Positive Psychology framework. *Journal of Deaf Studies and Deaf Education, 21*(3), 249–258.

Utami, D. S. (2018). *Life quality of families: Parenting issues, well-being profiles, and structural relationships among families of deaf or hard-of-hearing schoolchildren in Germany and Indonesia* (Unpublished doctoral dissertation). University of Leipzig, Leipzig.

World Health Organization (WHO). (2017, February). Deafness and hearing loss. Retrieved on December 20, 2017 from http://www.who.int/mediacentre/factsheets/fs300/en/

Zaidman-Zait, A. (2014, October 1). *Parenting stress among parents of deaf and hard-of-hearing children* (Electronic Bulletins). Retrieved on November 15, 2017 from http://www.raisingandeducatingdeafchildren.org/2014/10/01/parenting-stress-among-parents-of-deaf-and-hard-of-hearing-children

Zaidman-Zait, A., Most, T., Tarrasch, R., Haddad-eid, E., & Brand, D. (2016). The impact of childhood hearing loss on the family: Mothers' and fathers' stress and coping resources. *Journal of Deaf Studies and Deaf Education, 21*(1), 23–33.

Gunendra R. K. Dissanayake

# Most Frequent and Distressing Forms of Intimate Partner Psychological Abuse among Women in Sri Lankan Context

**Abstract:** Researchers have reported that psychological abuse is related to increased vulnerability to some clinical issues including psychological distress. A cross-sectional study was conducted to examine women related to increased vulnerability to some clinical issues including psychological distress. The survey was conducted with a sample of 200, 18–49-year-old help-seeking ever-partnered women. Pre-tested self-administered questionnaires assessing psychological abuse and psychological distress were the main instruments of data collection. Multiple regression analyzes revealed that psychological abuse contributed uniquely to the prediction of psychological distress, over and above the impact of physical and sexual abuse. Most frequent forms of psychological abuse reported by women were the woman experiencing the partner using money or making critical financial decisions without talking to her about it, partner blaming the woman for his problems, and not letting the woman talk about her feelings. As predicted, some forms of psychological abuse appeared more damaging than others. Specifically, ridiculing, ignoring, isolating, controlling, verbal harassment, threatening, manipulating, and non-supportive behavior emerged as the most distress causing forms of psychological abuse among the participants. Frequent forms of abuse were not necessarily the worst forms of abuse which exerted the most detrimental impact on women's psychological well-being. Clinicians should make the differentiation between most frequent and severe forms of psychological abuse when working with the clients. With the application of these results, counselling methods can be refined and tested for countering forms of abuse that cause the most lingering effects on psychological well-being.

**Keywords:** intimate partner violence, psychological abuse, Sri Lanka

## 1 Introduction

Studies exploring IPV, however, seem to have mainly focused on the effects of physical abuse, which is considered potentially life-threatening, overlooking the nature and effects of psychological abuse (Baldry, 2003; O'Leary, 1999). Psychological abuse, however, is found to exert a toll on victims that is just as damaging as physical abuse, if not more so than that of physical abuse (Follingstad, Rutledge, Berg, Hause, & Polek, 1990; Outlaw, 2009; Street & Arias, 2001). With the recognition of the devastating nature and effects of psychological abuse in intimate relations, there seems to be an advancement of studies researching this area. However, relatively little is known about the nature, different types and impact of psychological abuse among Asian women, especially Sri Lankan. Thus, as in Sri Lanka no published research studies have attempted to explore this critical issue so far, the objectives of the present study were to identify the most frequent forms of psychological abuse, and to determine the impact of various kinds of psychological abuse on the mental health well-being of the abused women.

## 2 Theoretical Review

Psychological abuse can be defined as recurring incidents of criticism, verbal abuse, and acts of domination and isolation that lead to control of the woman (O'Leary, 1999).

Researchers have reported that psychological abuse is related to increased vulnerability to a number of clinical issues including psychological distress, low self-esteem, substance abuse, cognitive impairment, depression and anxiety (Arias & Pape, 1999; Baldry, 2003; Hennings & Klesges, 2003; Ovara, McLeod, & Sharpe, 1996; Marshall, 1999). Further, it has been suggested that various forms of psychological abuse may not have similar effects on abused women showing that some types of psychological abuse appear more damaging than others (Chan, 2006; Follingstad et al., 1990; Sackett & Saunders, 2001; Tiwari, Chan, Fong, et al., 2008). The most frequent forms of psychological abuse might not be necessarily the worst forms carrying the most damaging effects. Thus, determining particular types of psychological abuse that cause more severe impacts is necessary to identify women who are at a higher risk of developing more detrimental consequences, and to modify and redefine counselling methods, and initiate intervention accordingly.

## 3 Method

### 3.1 Sample

The sample consisted of 200 ever-partnered women between 18 to 49 years. All the participants were help-seeking women, and they were randomly selected from ten women in help centres of five districts in Sri Lanka.

### 3.2 Measurement Tools

#### 3.2.1 *Psychological Maltreatment of Women Inventory (PMWI; Tolman, 1989)*

PMWI is a self-report instrument which asks the participant to rate each item on 5-response Likert scale. PMWI-long version which contains 58 items of two factor-derived subscales that measure dominance and isolation and emotional, verbal, monitoring abuse was used in the present study. The scale was adapted and validated in the Sri Lankan context before using in the present study. Cronbach's Alpha for this scale for the current study was 0.94.

### 3.2.2 Questionnaire on General Health (QGH)

WHO developed SRQ-20 as a screening tool to measure psychological distress and used it to assess mental health. Cronbach's Alpha for the QGH was 0.90.

## 3.3 Procedure

The present study was designed and conducted adhering to the WHO's ethical guidelines for doing research into "violence against women" (WHO, 2001). Before conducting the study, ethical approval was obtained from the ethics review board of the University of Colombo, Sri Lanka. Trained research assistants carried out the data collection in different locations.

# 4 Results

## 4.1 Characteristics of the Participants ($n$ = 200)

### 4.2

Out of the total number ($n$ = 200) of women who participated in the cross-sectional survey on psychological abuse against women by their intimate partners, (78%) were married, 1.5% were divorced, 1.5% were living together, and another 19% were separated. Age range varying between 20 to 49 years, mean age of the respondents was 34.22 ($SD$ = 7.50). Eighty-eight per cent (88%) of the women reported receiving a secondary level of education, whereas only a minority of women reported receiving primary (6%) and tertiary levels (6%).

## 4.3 Prevalence of IPV

Majority of the women in the sample (79%) reported being subjected to all three forms (psychological, physical and sexual) of abuse. All participants (100%) reported experiencing psychological abuse, whereas 96% and 81% of the participants reported being subjected to physical and sexual abuse consequently. Results of the study clearly show the co-occurrence of the multiple forms of abuse.

## 4.4 Nature of Psychological Abuse

The PMWI inventory used a six-point Likert-type response scale ranging from "Never" to "Not Applicable", the option not applicable being not scored. The forms of psychological abuse (with the highest mean scores) the respondents reported as 'frequently being subjected to', such as: "My partner used our money or made important financial decisions without talking to me about it" ($M$ = 4.43) with

Table 1. Most Frequent Forms of Psychological Abuse among the Respondents

| Most Frequent Forms of Psychological Abuse | M [a] | SD | Frequency in the past six months[a] (%) | | | | | | Response[b] |
|---|---|---|---|---|---|---|---|---|---|
| | | | 1 | 2 | 3 | 4 | 5 | NA[c] | |
| My partner used our money or made important financial decisions without talking to me about it | 4.43 | 1.00 | 2.5 | 4.0 | 5.5 | 21.5 | 66.0 | 0.5 | F |
| My partner blamed me for his problems | 4.37 | 0.83 | 0.5 | 3.5 | 9.0 | 32.5 | 54.5 | 0 | F |
| My partner said something to spite me | 4.36 | 0.83 | 1.0 | 3.5 | 6.5 | 36.5 | 52.5 | 0 | F |
| My partner did not let me talk about my feelings | 4.31 | 0.86 | 2.0 | 2.5 | 6.5 | 40.5 | 48.5 | 0 | F |
| My partner withheld affection from me | 4.28 | 0.87 | 0.5 | 4.5 | 11.0 | 34.5 | 49.5 | 0 | F |
| My partner blamed me when he was upset | 4.22 | 0.98 | 2.5 | 5.0 | 9.5 | 34.0 | 49.0 | 0 | F |
| My partner swore at me. | 4.21 | 0.97 | 1.0 | 7.0 | 11.5 | 31.5 | 49.0 | 0 | F |
| My partner acted irresponsibly with our financial resources. | 4.18 | 1.22 | 7.0 | 5.5 | 9.0 | 20.0 | 58.5 | 0 | F |

Notes. [a]Mean values based on the response scale 0 = Not Applicable, 1 = Never, 2 = Rarely, 3 = Occasionally, 4 = Frequently, 5 = Very frequently; [b]Response categories based on the following scale established by the researcher: < 1.51 = N-Never; 1.51 to 2.50 = R-Rarely; 2.51 to 3.50 = O-Occasionally; 3.51 to 4.50 = F-Frequently; >4.51 = VF-Very frequently; NA[c] stands for the option Not Applicable.

97% of the respondents reported experiencing some degree of this form of abuse, "My partner blamed me for his problems" ($M = 4.37$) with 99.5% reporting being subjected to this form, and "My partner said something to spite me" ($M = 4.36$) with 99% reporting to have experienced some degree of this form of abuse. Also included in the category of frequent forms of abuse were "My partner did not let me talk about my feelings" ($M = 4.31$) with 98% reporting experiencing some degree of this form of abuse and "My partner withheld affection from me" ($M = 4.28$) with 99.5% reported being subjected to some degree of this form of abuse. The mean response to each of these five items was classified in the "Frequently" response category. The most frequent forms of psychological abuse based on the mean response of each item is presented in Table 1.

## 4.5 Least Frequent Forms of Psychological Abuse

The study also examined the least frequent forms of psychological abuse. The forms of psychological abuse that reported by the respondents as 'least frequently being subjected to' include the items "My partner was jealous of other men", "My partner did not allow me to work", and "My partner tried to convince me and the others around me that I was crazy". These items had the mean scores falling in the 'Occasionally' category indicating that the respondents have not frequently experienced these behaviors.

## 4.6 Impact of Psychological Abuse on Psychological Distress

Psychological distress was significantly associated with increased levels of psychological abuse ($r(200) = 0.25$, $p < 0.01$), indicating that when the level of psychological abuse increased, level of psychological distress also increased. Multiple regression analysis, which examined the specific contribution of each form of psychological abuse in predicting psychological distress, revealed that some forms of psychological abuse exert more severe impacts. Controlling and isolating behaviors (My partner demanded to stay home and look after kids ($\beta = 0.33$, $p < 0.01$); My partner didn't allow to leave the house ($\beta = -0.39$, $p < 0.001$)) significantly contributed to the variance in psychological distress. Ridiculing forms of abuse such a treating the woman as stupid ($\beta = 0.45$, $p < 0.001$), insulting or shaming in front of others ($\beta = -0.22$, $p < 0.05$), and putting down the woman's physical appearance ($\beta = -0.19$, $p < 0.05$) also significantly contributed to the variance in psychological distress. Insensitive behavior including being insensitive to the woman's feelings ($\beta = -0.23$, $p < 0.05$) and being insensitive to sexual needs and desires ($\beta = 0.39$, $p < 0.05$) too added significantly to the variance in psychological distress. In addition, trying to convince the woman that she is crazy (My partner told me my feelings were irrational or crazy ($\beta = 0.23$, $p < 0.05$)), verbal abuse (My partner said something to spite me ($\beta = 0.27$, $p < 0.05$)), (My partner screamed and yelled ($\beta = -0.38$, $p < 0.05$)), blaming (Blamed for causing his violent behavior ($\beta = 0.30$, $p < 0.01$)), and threatening to take away kids ($\beta = -0.28$, $p < 0.01$) significantly contributed to the variance in psychological distress.

# 5 Conclusion

One of the objectives of the present study was to discover the frequent forms of psychological IPV in which the women in the Sri Lankan context were subjected. In the WHO multi-country study (2005) on domestic violence, the acts most frequently mentioned by women were insults, belittling and intimidation, whereas in Sri Lanka partner using money and making important financial decisions without consulting the woman, blaming and hurting were the most frequent forms. Hence, there appears to be a difference in some various forms of psychological abuse experienced by Sri Lankan women compared to countries included in the WHO multi-country study. However, findings of the study also show that some forms of psychological abuse the Sri Lankan women were subjected to are similar to those that other studies and conceptualisations also have reported. For example, the reported forms of psychological abuse in the current study are similar to the conceptualizations of psychological abuse presented by Tolman (1999), Murphy and Hoover (1999), and are consistent with the findings of Follingstad et al. (1990), Sackett and Saunders (2001), and Shuk-ting (2013).

The frequently forms of psychological abuse the women reported experiencing did not mean, however, that these forms of abuse necessarily were the worst forms of abuse which exerted the most detrimental impact on women's psychological well-being. For example, although being a frequent form of psychological IPV, experiencing the partner using money or making critical financial decisions without talking to the woman about it was not significantly associated with the level of psychological distress of the abused woman. It could be that, when living in a patriarchal society where men get the upper hand, women are used to men performing the decision making role and handling financial matters without consulting them. Hence, these forms of abuse might not generate much distress in the woman in the current context. However, there were some forms of abuse that women considered as worse than other forms which also lead to greater level of distress. These findings confirm the previous research which reveals that some types of psychological abuse exert more severe impacts than others (Sackett & Saunders, 1999; Tiwari et al., 2008). Confirming the previous findings (Aguilar & Nightingale, 1994), specifically, ridiculing, ignoring, isolating, controlling, verbal harassment, threatening, manipulating, and non-supportive behavior emerged as the most damaging forms of psychological abuse among the participants. Ridiculing forms of abuse, such as putting down the woman's physical appearance, insulting or shaming in front of others including trying to convince her and others around her that she is crazy, and treating the woman as stupid was strongly related to psychological distress. Previous research also has shown ridicule as the most destructive form of abuse when compared with jealousy, restriction, threats of abuse, and threats of divorce and damage to property (Follingstad et al., 1990). It can be assumed because acts that directly targeted in attacking a person's inner self would cause more distress than other types or forms of abuse. This finding is consistent with reports of abused women describing ridiculing behaviors as particularly pernicious (Follingstad et al., 1990; Sackett & Saunders, 1999). Ignoring was another form of abuse which was strongly related to psychological distress and feelings of self-worth. Previous research (e.g., Sackett & Saunders, 1999) also has shown that ignoring as one main types of psychological abuse most significantly related to depression.

Controlling, and isolating behaviors such as "My partner interfered in my relationships with other family members", "My partner didn't allow to leave the house", also were significantly related to psychological distress. Previously, Coker et al. (2002) use data from a national survey and conclude that abuse of power and control were more strongly predictive of depression rather than verbal abuse.

Considering the importance of these abusive forms, and the significance of controlling and restriction of recourses in the prediction of psychological distress, further research could clarify the importance of this particular form of abuse to the extended field and could have even wider implications for educating providers on how to assess a client's needs properly. Other forms of psychological abuse which were associated significantly with psychological distress were verbal abuse (e.g., "My partner said something to spite me", "My partner screamed and yelled") and blaming (e.g., "Blamed for causing his violent behavior"). These forms of abuse might be distress causing as these forms also are targeted towards one's internal self directly. To clarify this further, acts such as name-calling was not significant, despite this being a common example of psychological abuse. For practitioners, these findings confirm the negative impact the psychological abuse has the abused woman's emotional life and sense of self. Practitioners can help the abused women to see why some forms of psychological abuse are more damaging and distress causing than other forms of psychological abuse. With the replication of these results, counselling methods can be refined and tested for countering what forms of abuse probably cause the most lingering effects of psychological abuse-those which affect the survivor's very sense of self.

# 6 Affiliation

Dr. Gunendra R. K. Dissanayake
Institution: University of Peradeniya, Sri Lanka.
Address: Department of Philosophy and Psychology, University of Peradeniya, Peradeniya, 20400.
E-mail: asabhakeeragala@gmail.com, gunendrad@pdn.ac.lk

# 7 References

Aguilar, R. J., & Nightingale, N. N. (1994). The impact of specific battering experiences on the self-esteem of abused women. *Journal of Family Violence, 9*(1), 35–45.

Arias, I., & Pape, K. T. (1999). Psychological abuse: Implications for adjustment and commitment to leave violent partners. *Violence and Victims, 14*(1), 55–67.

Baldry, A. C. (2003). Sticks and stones hurt my bones but his glance and words hurt more: The impact of psychological abuse and physical violence by former and current partners on battered women in Italy. *International Journal of Forensic Mental Health, 2*, 47–57.

Chan, K. L. (2006). The Chinese concept of face and violence against women. *International Social Work, 49*(1), 65–73.

Coker, A. L., Smith, P. H., Thompson, M. P., McKeown, R. E., Bethea, L., & Davis, K. E. (2002). Social support protects against the negative effects of partner violence on mental health. *Journal of Women's Health and Gender-Based Medicine, 11,* 465–476.

Follingstad, D. R., Rutledge, L. L., Berg, B. J., Hause, E. S., & Ploek, D. S. (1990). The role of emotional abuse in physical abusive relationships. *Journal of Family Violence, 5,* 107–120.

Hennings, K. R., & Klesges, L. M. (2003). Prevalence and characteristics of psychological abuse reported by court involved battered women. *Journal of Interpersonal Violence, 18,* 857–871.

Marshall, L. L. (1999). Effects of men's subtle and overt psychological abuse on low-income women. *Violence and Victims, 14*(1), 69–88.

Murphy, C. M., & Hoover, S. A. (1999). Measuring emotional abuse in dating relationships as a multifactorial construct. *Violence and Victims, 14,* 39–53.

O'Leary, K. D. (1999). Psychological abuse: A variable deserving critical attention in domestic violence. *Violence and Victims, 14,* 3–23.

Ovara, T. A., McLeod, P. J., & Sharpe, D. (1996). Perception of control, depressive symptomatology and self-esteem of women in transition from abusive relationships. *Journal of Family Violence, 11,* 167–186.

Sackett, L. A., & Saunders, D. G. (2001). The impact of different forms of psychological abuse on battered women. In K. D. O'Leary & R. D. Maiuro (Eds.), *Psychologica abuse in violent domestic relations* (pp. 197–210). New York: Springer.

Shuk-ting. (2013). *Validation of the psychological maltreatment of women inventory for Chinese women* (Unpublished master thesis). University of Hong Kong, Hong Kong.

Street, A. E., & Arias, I. (2001). Psychological abuse and posttraumatic stress disorder in battered women: examining the roles of shame and guilt. *Violence and Victims, 16,* 65–78.

Tiwari, A., Chan, K., Fong, D., Leung, W., Brownridge, D., Lam, H., … Ho, P. (2008). The impact of psychological abuse by an intimate partner on the mental health of pregnant women. *BJOG An International Journal of Obstetrics and Gynaecology, 115*(3), 377–84.

Tolman, R. M. (1999). The validation of the psychological maltreatment of women inventory. *Violence and Victims, 14*(1), 25–35.

World Health Organization. (2001). *Putting women first: Ethical and safety recommendations for research on domestic violence against women,* WHO/FCH/GWH/01.1. Retrieved on September 2, 2017 from http://apps.who.int/iris/bitstream/handle/10665/65893/WHO_FCH_GWH_01.1.pdf.

World Health Organization. (2005). *WHO Multi-Country Study on Women's Health and Domestic Violence against Women* (Summary Report). Geneva, Switzerland: Author.

Emi Zulaifah, Hazhira Qudsyi, Rumiani, & Sri Wahyuningsih

# Strategies for Controlling Internet Usage in Dual-Earner Families

**Abstract:** The wider uses of internet access among various age segments in Indonesia become the main trigger in our attempt to understand the pattern of internet usage in families. It begins with a concern that besides the benefits of the widely available access, the internet can also bring disadvantages, especially for the minor family members. At the same time, it becomes urgent that the pattern of usage and the need for controlling the access as well as the strategies that family can employ are known for the wiser use of internet access. The dual career families were chosen as our cases, based on the fact that without the challenge of controlling the internet, such families are already faced with work-family interface issues. Thus the situation can become more difficult with internet access as part of the family matters to handle. This study used a qualitative approach, with multiple case studies design. The participants were family members (6 parents) and one family member who is an excessive online gamer. All participants have faced challenges in managing control for Internet usage. Four themes that cover the pattern of usage and misuse of online access were identified, namely: Patterns of usage and misuse, the impact of excessive and prolonged usage, strategies for control of internet access, and factors contributing to an effective strategy.

**Keywords:** internet access in families, internet controls strategies

## 1 Introduction

The ministry of information released the current data on internet usage (Kominfo, 2017). At least 30 million children and youths in Indonesia are internet user, and digital media are the chosen media of communication that young people of today have widely accepted. In fact, one of the purposes of development in Indonesia is to create wider accessibility of the internet, and by 2015 this goal is achieved by 50% of Indonesian populations wired online (BAPPENAS [National Development Agency], 2007). The results of one study by the Indonesian Ministry of Information, United Nations Children's Fund (UNICEF) and Harvard University, using 400 youths ages 10 to 19 from 11 provinces around Indonesia revealed that 80% surveyed respondents were internet users. In Yogyakarta, Jakarta, and Banten for example, the respondents were all internet users. While in other areas such as West Papua and Northern Moluccas less than 1/3 of the respondents were internet users. This fact shows that there is a huge digital divide between areas in Java and remote Islands of Indonesia. This is a worldwide phenomenon as noted by International Telecommunication Union [ITU] (Livingstone, 2014) that

Table 1. Negative internet experience among youths in Indonesia

| Negative Internet Experiences | N | Percentage |
|---|---|---|
| Connect with strangers | 96 | 24% |
| Cyber bullying | 52 | 13% |
| Inappropriate sexual content | 56 | 14% |

*Noted. N = number of participants;* N Total = 400, only problematic internet uses are listed in the table.

the percentage of internet access is 41% of the world population and 28% of the population is in the developing world. With such a vast number of young people accessing online information from around the world, which often unfiltered, Livingstone (2014) underlined that it is not very easy to imagine the impacts of the ease of access and the use of the internet that involve very young age in such enormous scope. Further data on internet usage among youngsters in Indonesia also showed that they misused internet as shown in Table 1 as the negative internet experiences.

The National Commission of Children Protection/KPAI (Republika, 2014) researched by using 300 respondents of elementary school pupils from 4th to 6th grade and found that 62% of them were exposed to the internet with inappropriate sexual content. Data in the National Commission of Children Protection (Republika, 2014) revealed that maltreatment towards children is often triggered by the perpetrators as a result of learning from the internet the wrong way. With children becoming the major concern, it is of no surprise that in fact over 45 million Indonesian adults access much sexual content on the internet. Misused of internet access, thus, have resulted in unanticipated impacts, wide in scope and varied in ages. The data in Figure 1 is the findings from a short study through various national online media, examining the news for (only) extreme cases from the year 2010 to 2017 that are triggered by online media access. It revealed the following results:

Today, the Indonesian government has decreed that murder, sexual assault and death triggered by online access are considered as extraordinary crimes. The National Commissions of Children Protection have repeatedly underlined the critical roles of families in guarding the interactions between its members with the online virtual world. The current study is responding to these issues.

The purpose of this study is to 1) Understand in depth the use of the internet both in the advantage and disadvantage sides and the need to control its usage; 2) The impact of the misused and excessive online access; and 3) The strategies employed in order to have effective control over internet access and identify factors that contribute to the wise use of Internet.

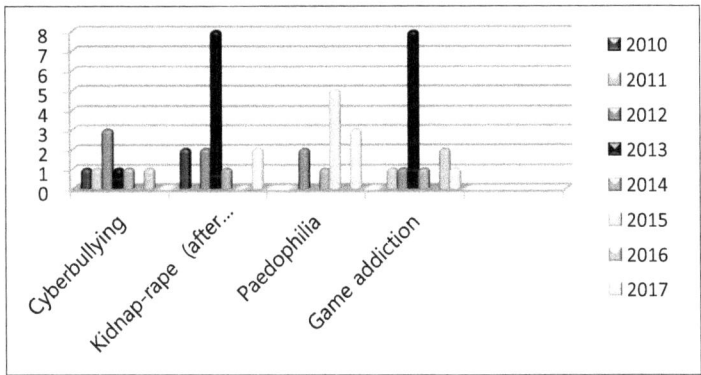

**Figure 1.** Further consequences of the misuse of online access

*Information for figure 1: Category I: Cyberbullying; Category II: Kidnap-rape (after social media contact); Category III: Paedophilia; Category IV: Game addiction. Most categories of problematic online access are self explanatory. However, cyberbullying might need to be described. According to KidsHealth (2014) cyberbullying is the use of technology to harass, threaten, embarrass, or target another person. By definition, it occurs among young people.*

## 2 Theoretical Review

Comprehensive research studies on the benefits of internet access were in fact carried out in the area of learning and instructional technology. Some of them were done in the USA (Rideout, 2014; Harvard Family Research Project [HFRP], 2014) and assumed that digital media, including the use of the internet would benefit learning. This area of research did not identify the mechanism in which internet benefit can be maximized and the negative impact is put into its minimum level. A study from Psychology and the media showed otherwise the negative impact of internet usage. Such disadvantages are identified as follow: the less time for personal communication, increase of depression and loneliness (Hughes, Ebata, & Dollahite, 1999; Kraut, Patterson, Lundmark, Kiesler, Mukophadhyay, & Scherlis, 1998; Stanford Institute for the Quantitative Study of Society, 2000). A more recent study, however, revealed otherwise different results, such as more connection with friends through the internet (Gross, 2004). Support from parents during internet access will increase the likelihood of accessing educational information (Lee & Chae, 2007), although cases of internet addiction drove therapist to come with intervention such as through CBT (Young, 2007). This means that, nonetheless, the promising side of Internet access still needs to be critically viewed as cases of problematic Internet use do take place. The challenges faced by Indonesian families in dealing with Internet use are not yet well understood, after the facts that misused of the internet have led to various unwanted shocking and often traumatic events such as found in the online news data above.

## 3 Method

### 3.1 Study participants

This study is the first step of a longitudinal study on strategies of controlling internet usage. The participant of the preliminary study is one online gamer and six parents (working mothers) who have to deal with children accessing the internet in their early childhood and those who provide internet access for their teenagers. The participants' criteria were determined as such to allow for the examination of the experience of online access, and strategies developed for effective control within different age groups.

### 3.2 Data collection method

Data were collected using in-depth interview. With the online gamer, a repeated interview was done for further clarification of some of his statement from the first interview. With the six parents, the interviews were conducted once for each with the possibility of clarifying their statement at any time needed. Observations were done during the interview and on different occasions. The interview protocol was initially developed to include the following questions: 1) What are the reasons to provide Internet access in the family? 2) What kinds of usage are present after the available access? 3) What will normally trigger the need to access? 4) The experiences – the advantages of having the access and the disadvantages? 5) In their experience, what kind of impact are present that they can observe in family members, this could be the positive or negative impact? 6) Given that family members varies in ages and as access can be misused, what are the strategies employed by the family to control its usage?

## 4 Results

Following the qualitative tradition stated by Merriam and Tisdell (2016), our data analysis is done firstly through open coding and then followed by categorisation into units of meanings. Through the process, we identified four categories of themes, namely: pattern of use and misuse, the impact of excessive usage, strategies to control Internet usage, and factors contributing to effective strategies, each with subcategories.

### 4.1 Pattern of Use and Misuse

*The ease of information seeking, learning and communicating* mark the beginning of access provided in the household. Almost all respondents agreed that this is the main reason why online access is deemed necessary within the family.

*The onset of attachment to the internet*: Attachment to the internet does not occur without a beginning. It is interesting that various ways are found on how children (and continued into their teens) become attached to using the Internet. *Modelling from parents, older family members and peers* serve as the direct mechanism on how children get attached to the internet, especially through gadgets, often before children are not yet in school. Children are interested in the tool after seeing parents, and older family members are using them, and seeing their peer at play, the young children often bring with them gadgets to play together. Another factor that brings children to the Internet more intensively comes from the school, starting from the beliefs that the *internet is a useful resource for education* that circulated and practised among schoolteachers. School assignments are often done with the Internet as the media for searching for the information. Without parental control, the intended schoolwork could lead to other uses that are not related to assignments.

One attribute that occurs with the online access that tends to be misused/problematic is excessive and prolonged access. All parents stated that lengthy access occur because parents tend to get busy with other things and leave the children with their device. Internet access could go rather out of control, especially for children, when they started learning about the fun application, such as watching movies (cartoon) in YouTube or game application that can be downloaded freely. Thus, misuse of the internet could start very early in childhood. Often, parents give the gadget to keep the children quiet in order not to disturb their engagement in one activity.

### 4.2 Impact of Excessive and Prolonged Usage

As an attachment to intensive access of internet occurs, it becomes more challenging for parents to detach children from it, leading the way to excessive and prolonged Internet use. Usually, acts of protest such as through expressed anger and temper-tantrums (negative emotions) will indicate that they are upset when detached. All parents agree that such access is always possible and that occasions of accessing inappropriate content happened. Meanwhile the impacts of excessive usage that also appear in the older youth can touch different areas, such as: health (fatigue, sleep disturbance), soft skill (inability to set priority such as choosing to play games over school class), limited social interaction (such as socializing more with the gamers community and less interested in other social activity) and academic (lower school grade). Cognitive preoccupation moderates the excessive use, Caplan and High (2006) found. This is something that we are interested in examining the impacts further among the excessive users. On the positive side, accessing internet intensively can help older youth to improve their study and task completion, such as through online video tutorial, and contacts and activity arrangements with friends are made more convenient. Overall, the excessive, prolonged use of the internet could lead to life imbalance if not handled properly and that purpose of access becomes the defining line whether the extensive and continued access will be beneficial or detrimental.

### 4.3 Strategies for control of Internet access

Parents do develop strategies to control online internet access. Some principles and practices are identified as the main strategy: Setting rules and apply conditions, such as through agreement on limiting time, quota and purpose of access and applying conditions of usage, such as not to forget homework. Alternative activities: parents stated that to distract their children from logging into the Internet too much is by giving them alternative activities. They admit that it becomes costly to get them engaged in other things, as it might involve going outdoors, buying more educational toys. For the strategy to be effective, a supporting strategy is developed, namely: dialogue, chaperoning, and rewards. Open dialogue is deemed important by parents as it allows them to convey essential messages regarding important values, such as: asking permission, using time wisely, and carefulness when it involved strangers. Chaperoning is done through being together with the children when the needs to access come. In this way, the explanation can be given on how things should be done, such as typing the right keywords for searching in order not to yield wrong links. This is in line with Lee and Chae's (2007) study in Korea that found parents' internet suggestion and co-using is associated with the children frequency of accessing educational websites. However, older youth dialogue is more often used and emphasized than chaperoning. With the dialogue, their youths find it easy to convey their experience through Internet browsing. The religious parents use dialogue to convey the critical principles relevant to usage of tools and man-made inventions.

The factors that contribute to the effectiveness of the strategy vary and can be identified as follow: Dispositional factor (some children are not easy in listening to their parents' advice and remain ignorant). On the other hand, the self-regulation part appeared as problematic when it comes to the excessive use of the Internet and inability to prioritise. Other dispositional factors also influence how things are communicated, such as trust (trusting that their children know what is expected), assertiveness (especially when rules are broken). Being internet savvy and parental role model: All parents believe that effective control is not made possible when they do not know much about the Internet (being savvy) or when there is absence of a role model (parents are good in telling, but they also need to show things they tell as right), thus acting as their role model for wise internet use is deemed ideal. For this, cohesion between the busy father and mother is much needed.

## 5 Discussion and Conclusion

The study was aimed at exploring how families are dealing with continues internet access within their household among family members. The four themes and subthemes found gave us a better understanding that the coming of information revolution does give effect to family interaction. Benefits are gained such as from the convenience of learning and communicating, yet some consequences need to be looked upon more carefully. Families (in this case are dual-earner, middle-class families in Indonesia) do show awareness of the challenges in handling Internet access in their household. Maximising its use for the beneficial sides is not always easy, in line with Gross (2004) statement as it involves multitasking, and – as found in the current study – need careful attention and the right strategy. What is not yet explored at this stage is whether or not attached to the internet will influence the social sensitivity, or empathy towards other people (Larson, 1995), and the keenness of the younger generation towards handling real-world problems. In making Indonesia better, we need people to be actively involved, engaged and to get their hands at work, not only browsing the Internet; this should warrant open-ended survey in further studies, to be able to portray Indonesian youths at large in their habit of internet usage.

# 6 Affiliations

Dr. Emi Zulaifah
Institution: Department of Psychology, Islamic University of Indonesia (UII)
Address: UII Main Campus, Jalan Kaliurang Km 14.5, Yogyakarta 55584, Indonesia.
E-mail: emiriyono@gmail.com

M. A. Hazhira Qudsyi
Institution: Department of Psychology, Islamic University of Indonesia (UII)
Address: UII Main Campus, Jalan Kaliurang Km 14.5, Yogyakarta 55584, Indonesia.
E-mail: hazhira.qudsyi@uii.ac.id

M. Psi. Rumiani
Institution: Department of Psychology, Islamic University of Indonesia (UII)
Address: UII Main Campus, Jalan Kaliurang Km 14.5, Yogyakarta 55584, Indonesia.
E-mail: rumiani@uii.ac.id

S. Psi. Sri Wahyuningsih
Institution: Department of Psychology, Islamic University of Indonesia
Address: UII Main Campus, Jalan Kaliurang Km 14.5, Yogyakarta 55584, Indonesia.
E-mail: sri.wahyuningsih@ymail.com

# 7 References

Bappenas. (2007). *Laporan Perkembangan Pencapaian Millennium Development Goals, Indonesia 2007*. Jakarta: Ministry of National Development Planning Indonesia.

Caplan S. E., & High, A. C. (2006). Beyond excessive use: The interaction between cognitive and behavioral symptoms of problematic internet use. *Communication Research Reports, 23*(4), 265–271.

Gross, E. F. (2004). Adolescent internet use: What we expect, what teens report. *Applied Developmental Psychology, 25*, 633–649.

Harvard Family Research Project. (2014). *Families and digital media in Young Children's learning*. Retrieved on January 15, 2018 from http://www.hfrp.org/var/hfrp/storage/fckeditor/File/HFRP_ResearchSpotlight_Families_and_Digital_Media021914.pdf

Hughes, R., Ebata, A. T., & Dollahite, D. C. (1999). Family life in the information age. *Family Relations, 48,* 5–6.

KidsHealth (2014). *Cyberbullying.* Retrived on January 15, 2018 from https://kidshealth.org/en/parents/cyberbullying.html

Kominfo. (2014). *Press release: Kominfo and UNICEF's research on children and youth behavior in Internet usage.* Retrieved on February 5, 2018 from https://kominfo.go.id/content/detail/3834/siaran-pers-no-17pihkominfo22014-tentang-riset-kominfo-dan-unicef-mengenai-perilaku-anak-dan-remaja-dalam-menggunakan-internet/0/siaran_pers

Kraut, R., Patterson, M., Lundmark, V., Kiesler, S., Mukophadhyay, T., & Scherlis, W. (1998). Internet paradox: A social technology that reduces social involvement and psychological well-being? *American Psychologist, 53,* 1017–1031.

Larson, R. W. (1995). Secrets in the bedroom: Adolescents' private use of media. *Journal of Youth and Adolescence, 24,* 535–550.

Lee, S. J., & Chae, Y. G. (2007). Children's internet use in a family context: Influence on family relationships and parental mediation. *Cyberpsychology & Behavior, 10*(5). doi: 10.1089/cpb.2007.9975

Livingstone, S. (2014). Children's digital rights: A priority. *Intermedia, 42*(4), 20–24.

Merriam, S. B., & Tisdell, E. J. (2016). *Qualitative research: A guide to design and implementation* (4th edition). San Francisco: John Wiley & Sons, Inc.

Republika. (2014). *62 Persen Anak SD Kecanduan Pornografi* [62 Percent children are porn addicts]. Retrieved on February 5, 2018 from http://nasional.republika.co.id/berita/nasional/Umum/14/06/21/n7i49e-62-persen-anak-sd-kecanduan-pornografi

Rideout, V. J. (2014). *Learning at home: Families' educational media use in America: A report of the families and media project.* New York: The Joan Ganz Cooney Center at Sesame Workshop.

Stanford Institute for the Quantitative Study of Society. (2000). *Study offers early look at how Internet is changing daily life (Press Release).* Retrieved on February 2, 2018 from http://standford.edu/dept/news/pr/00/000216Internet.html

Young, K. (2007). Cognitive behavior therapy with Internet addicts: Treatment outcomes and implication. *Cyber Psychology and Behavior, 10*(5). doi: 10.1089/cpb.2007.9975

Bagus Riyono & Annisa Rizkiayu Leofianti

# The Role of Social Support to Cope with Work-Family Conflict

**Abstract:** Family is a pivotal issue in social science following the policy of sustainable development that is established by the United Nations. In order for the society to be sustainable the well-being of families should be prioritised among other social issues. European countries have decided to implement family-friendly policy in order to foster family well-being and family sustainability. One of the threat to family well-being is work-family conflict as a result of the increasing working mothers. To bring mothers back to families is almost impossible in a short time, but reducing work-family conflict will be the reasonable steps to cope with the problems. This study investigates the role of social support to reduce work-family conflict. The study was conducted among female nurses in Yogyakarta, Indonesia. Data was collected with two questionnaires to measure the intensity of work-family conflict and the extent of social support from the spouse, the colleagues and from the superior. There were 70 subjects included in the study. The data was analyzed with stepwise Regression analysis with three predictors, i.e. spouse support, colleagues support, and superior support. The results showed that social support from colleagues is the strongest variable that significantly reduce work-to-family conflict with the standardised regression coefficient ($\beta$) of -0.293, $p < 0.05$. Path analysis was conducted to investigate the overall role of social support. It is discussed why the colleague support is the one that is the most significant to reduce work-to-family interference.

**Keywords:** sustainable development, work-family conflict, social support

## 1 Introduction

Family is a pivotal issue in social science following the policy of sustainable development that is established by the United Nations. For the society to be sustainable, the well-being of families should be prioritised among other social issues. However, women participation in the workforce is needed to create balance and to ensure the sufficiency of family income among the lower economic status families (Utting, 2013).

European countries have decided to implement family-friendly policy to foster family well-being and family sustainability. The European Policy Brief on Families and Societies (Neyer, Thévenon, & Monfardini, 2016) make six recommendations as follows: (1) A modern European family policy should be a coherent mix of measures that provides support to a diverse variety of families during their entire life courses across all European countries; (2) Policies preventing early school leaving and welfare policies that support youths directly (social assistance, housing, and education subsidies) should be promoted, instead of indirect benefits via their parents; (3) Countries should create policies allowing for greater job flexibility. The right of citizens to request flexible work is of crucial importance when pursuing work-life balance and gender equality; (4) Policies should ease it for parents to spend time with their children by providing generous and flexible parental leaves for both mothers and fathers; (5) EU-level regulations on leave options are of great importance in setting minimum standards, and in influencing entitlements, length, flexibility and payment levels to facilitate reaching the employment targets and the gender equality objective. In line with this, EU-regulation of paternity leave should not be postponed any further; (6) Governments need to invest in improving the provision and the quality of formal childcare on full- time basis also for children below age three, and to promote its use among families.

The study of family well-being across the history of Europe concluded that in the 1960s the European families were at the ideal state when most of the women were house mothers (Utting, 2013). One of the threats to family well-being is work-family conflict as a result of the increasing working mothers. To bring mothers back to families is almost impossible in a short time, but reducing work-family conflict will be the reasonable steps to cope with the problems. This study investigates the role of social support to reduce work-family conflict.

## 2 Literature

Work-family conflict refers to the extent to which work- and family-related responsibilities interfere with each other (Greenhaus & Beutell, 1985). It is a conflict of work and family interrelated roles. Work-family conflict occurs when contribution in work role creates problems in contribution of family role (Greenhaus & Beutell, 1985). It is also documented that work-family conflict could arise from tough time demands, stress originated in one role spill over to other role disturbing the quality of life, and behaviors that were appropriate in one domain but are considered as inappropriate in other domain (Sultana & Alam, 2012).

The study investigating the difference of stress level between working mother and non-working mothers in Malaysia showed that working mothers experience more stress due to the double role as a house mother and as a worker (Sultana & Alam, 2012). Most of working women are having stress related to heavy workload and time constraints that might lead to work-family conflict.

Senécal, Vallerand, and Guay (2001) investigated the model of work-family conflict involving social support as antecedence and emotional exhaustion as consequence. Using the Structural Equation Modelling analysis, the model is confirmed that social support from spouse and employers have significant contribution to reduce work-family conflict through reducing family alienation. Meanwhile, work-family conflict is significantly predicting emotional exhaustion.

Grant-Vallone and Donaldson (2001) studied the effects of work-family conflict across time toward the well-being of the employees and their co-workers. Through a longitudinal study, it was found that the impact of work-family conflict on the well-being of the employees and their co-workers are significantly negative. Work-family conflict has a negative impact even on the co-worker's well-being in the long run.

The literature review shows that work-family conflict is a serious issue that can damage the employee, the family and even the co-worker's well-being. It is imperative that the effort to prevent or at least reduce the work-family conflict has to be done continuously. Social support has been identified to be the important variable to reduce the work-family conflict. However, the previous study has not investigated the support from co-worker or colleague as the significant others that have more intensity in a day-to-day work relationship. Therefore, this study includes the colleague support as part of the social support variables that are hypothesised to have the role in reducing work-family conflict.

# 3 Method

## 3.1 Sample

The sample of this study is 70 female nurses working at local hospitals in Yogyakarta, Indonesia. All of them have young children and live with their husbands. The sample work at two different hospitals that represent public and private institutions.

## 3.2 Measurement Tools

This study uses two measurement tools in the form of questionnaires to measure the intensity of work-family conflict, and the amount of social support received from the spouse, the supervisor, and the colleagues.

### 3.2.1 *The Work-Family Conflict Questionnaire*

The Work-Family Conflict questionnaire is adapted from Carlson, Kacmar and Williams (2000). This questionnaire measure three aspects of the work-family conflict, i.e., time-based conflict (22 items), strain-based conflict (24 items), and behavioral based conflict (14 items). For each aspect, the conflict is measured in two directions, i.e., Work-to-Family Interference (WIF) and Family-to-Work Interference (FIW). For the aspect of time-based conflict and behavioral-based conflict, the number of items for WIF and FIW is a balance. For strain-based conflict, there are more items on the WIF side because work usually more demanding and create more strain.

### 3.2.2 *Social Support Questionnaire*

The Social Support questionnaire is adapted from Cohen and McKay (1984). This questionnaire includes three aspects of social support, i.e., material support, appraisal support and emotional support. For each aspect there are three sources of support, i.e., spouse, superior, and colleagues.

Table 1. Blue Print of the Work-Family Conflict Questionnaire

| Aspects | Indicators | Total items | Direction | |
|---|---|---|---|---|
| | | | WIF | FIW |
| Time-based conflict | Conflicting time allocation between family and job | 22 | 11 | 11 |
| Strain-based conflict | Conflicts as a result of stress on the job as well as in the family | 24 | 15 | 9 |
| Behavior-based conflict | The behavioral problem that is considered inappropriate either in the job or the family | 14 | 7 | 7 |

Note. WIF = Work Interfere Family. FIW = Family Interfere Work.

Table 2. Blue print of the Social Support Conflict Questionnaire

| Aspects | Indicators | Source | | |
|---|---|---|---|---|
| | | Spouse | Superior | Colleagues |
| Material Support | Tangible support, facilities | 5 | 5 | 5 |
| Appraisal support | Positive remarks | 5 | 5 | 5 |
| Emotional support | Shown empathy | 5 | 5 | 5 |

## 4 Results

The results of the zero-order correlations are as follows. Table 3 shows that overall social support is significantly negatively correlated with work-family conflict. However, the social support of spouse, superior and colleague are inter-correlated to each other.

The data was then analyzed with Stepwise Regression analysis to identify the most significant independent variables (social support) in predicting the dependent variable (work-family conflict). The results of the stepwise regression analysis showed that colleague support is the only remaining independent variable that predicts the intensity of work-family conflict, with the standardised regression coefficient $(\beta)$ = -.293, $p < .05$.

The path analysis that includes all independent variables resulted in a path diagram as shown in Figure 1. The model shows that all variable are significantly correlated with each other. Work-family conflict is negatively correlated with all social support variables. The colleague support has the strongest predictive

**Table 3.** Correlation matrix across variables

| Variables | Mean | SD | 1 | 2 | 3 |
|---|---|---|---|---|---|
| 1. Work-Family Conflict | 1.92 | .48 | - | | |
| 2. Spouse Support | 4.05 | .52 | -.253* | - | |
| 3. Superior Support | 3.80 | .45 | -.265* | .386** | - |
| 4. Colleague Support | 3.69 | .44 | -.293* | .403** | .479** |

Note. * $p<.05$. ** $p<.01$

**Table 4.** Results of Stepwise Regression Analysis

| Social Supports | t | p | ß | F | df | p | Adj. $R^2$ |
|---|---|---|---|---|---|---|---|
| Entered Variable | | | | | | | |
| Colleague Support | -2.53 | .014 | -.293 | 6.375 | 1 | .014 | .072 |
| Excluded Variables | | | | | | | |
| Superior Support | -1.226 | .224 | -.161 | | | | |
| Spouse Support | -1.278 | .206 | -.161 | | | | |

Note. The dependent variable is the Work-Family Conflict

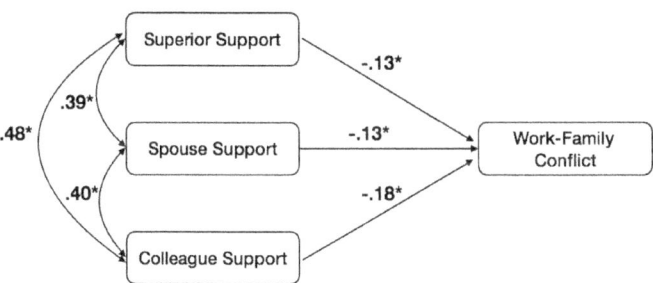

**Figure 1.** Path Model of Social Support and Work-to-Family Conflict

value ($ß = - 0.18$, $p < 0.05$). Both the superior support and spouse support has similar predictive value ($ß = - 0.13$, $p < 0.05$). Colleague support is highly correlated with superior support ($ß = 0.48$, $p < 0.05$) and spouse support ($ß = 0.40$, $p < 0.05$). While spouse support is also significantly correlated with superior support ($ß = 0.39$, $p < 0.05$).

## 5 Discussion

Colleague support is the most influential variable as the predictor of work-family conflict as the result of Stepwise Regression Analysis. This results support the hypothesis that colleague support has a significant role in reducing work-family conflict. This phenomenon is only logical since the most time spent in an employee work life is with their colleagues. This is even more relevant in the case of nurses. The path analysis confirmed that colleague support has a significant role besides spouse and superior support in reducing work-family conflict. Colleague support does not only add up to the role of spouse and superior support, but it is the most important one.

Based on the result of this study it is recommended for organizations that employ women to build a culture with the high quality of work life. Quality of work life is indicated by the quality of relationship among colleagues based on the values of trust, respect and care. These values represent the emotional support and appraisal support among colleagues. Even though material support is also essential, it is more the responsibility of the superior and spouse.

This study has confirmed the previous study about the important role of social support to reduce work-family conflict and add up with colleague support as the third dimension of social support.

## 6 Affiliations

Dr. Bagus Riyono
Institution: Faculty of Psychology, Universitas Gadjah Mada
Address: Jalan Sosio Humaniora No 1, Bulaksumur, Yogyakarta, Indonesia
E-mail: bagus@ugm.ac.id

Annisa Rizkiayu Leofianti
Institution: Faculty of Psychology, Universitas Gadjah Mada
Address: Jalan Sosio Humaniora No 1, Bulaksumur, Yogyakarta, Indonesia
E-mail: annisa.rizkiayu@ksp.go.id

## 7 References

Carlson, D. S., Kacmar, M. K., & Williams, L. J. (2000). Construction and validation of a multidimensional measure of work-family conflict. *Journal of Vocational Behavior, 56*(2), 249–276.

Cohen, S., & Mc.Kay, G. (1984). Social Support, Stress and the Buffering Hypothesis: A Theoretical Analysis. In S. E. T. Baum, & J. E. Singer. *Handbook of Psychology and Health* (pp. 253–267). New Jersey: Hillsdale.

Grant-Vallone, E. J., & Donaldson, S. I. (2001). Consequences of work-family conflict on employee well-being over time. *Work & Stress, 15* (3), 214–226.

Greenhaus, J. H., & Beutell, N. J. (1985). Source of conflict between work and family roles. *Academy of Management Review, 10*, 76–88.

Neyer, G., Thévenon, O., & Monfardini, C. (2016). *European Policy Brief on Family and Societies.* Max Planck Society for the Advancement of Science/Population Europe.

Senécal, C., Vallerand, R.J., & Guay, F. (2001). Antecedents and outcomes of work-family conflict: toward a motivational model. *Personality and Social Psychology Bulletin, 27*(2), 176–186.

Sultana, A. M., & Alam, Md. F. (2012). A study on stress and work-family conflict among married women in their families. *Journal of Applied Sciences Research, 8*(8), 4161–4166.

Utting, P. (2013). Revisiting sustainable development. *UNRISD Classics Vol. III.* Geneva: United Research Institute for Social Development.

# Chapter 3   Dyslexia

Evelin Witruk

# Dyslexia – Does It Still Exist?

**Abstract:** This contribution will give an overview of methods of assessment and intervention of dyslexia that focus on children. By the multilevel model, the methods of assessment and intervention could be ordered. On this way we find out new, alternative methods for assessment and intervention, and discuss these together.

**Keywords:** dyslexia, assessment, intervention methods, alternative new methods

## 1 Introduction

This contribution aims to find out an answer to the question about dyslexia, whether it still exists. My contribution will show examples of our dyslexia research from the last twenty years, and I am feeling very good to be supported by experts from the whole world.

The traditional approaches are related to theoretical hypotheses about a supposed deficit and try to measure and assess this with the aim to reduce or eliminate the deficit. The alternative new methods try to find out and measure the resources or strengths of a dyslexic individual and use these as a basis of intervention or prevention.

The different prevalence rates of dyslexia in the world varied from 1% in Scandinavian countries; 2% around the region of Beijing, Greece, and Spain; 3–5% in Germany; 8–10% in United Kingdom, United States of America, Morocco and Hong Kong; and leads to the question of the cultural or language impact on the development of dyslexia in a specific language or cultural environment.

## 2 Dyslexia Assessment Methods

In the multilevel-model, the assessment methods are ordered after focus on the achievement of the primary and secondary reasons. That means the method can be started on the assessment of biological risk factors like the genetic code or the factors of the phonological or visual persistence. From this basis, these partial performance deficits begin its development, and it can be measured until the end of the kindergarten time. On this level, we can find the specific deficiencies in the working memory as found in comparing with dyslexic children from Hong Kong (Witruk, 2017).

On the level of primary symptoms, a lot of reading and writing tests are developed. The diagnosis "Dyslexia" is earliest from the end of first grade possible when the intelligence is in the normal region. From this stage, we can find a development of secondary symptoms like anxiety, aggression or depression. We could compare

Table 1. Multilevel model with assessment and intervention methods

|  |  | Assessment | Intervention |
|---|---|---|---|
| Reasons | Primary | Biological risk factors | Compensatory training |
|  | Secondary | Partial performance deficits | Training of basic functions, prevention |
| Symptoms | Primary | Reading and writing tests | Rehabilitative exercises and training programs for reading |
|  | Secondary | Personality questionnaires, observations | Complex training, psychotherapy |

the secondary symptoms of dyslexics in Indonesia, Morocco and Germany (Novita, 2015; Raziq, 2008) and could see the impact of culture on the development of these secondary symptoms.

## 3 Dyslexia Intervention Methods

In the multilevel-model, the intervention methods are ordered in the same way dependence on their relevance and lifetime of their application. When there is a child with high biological risk factors (father was and is a dyslexic individual) then it can done through an exercise through kinesiological training with the kindergarten-children (Dennison & Dennison, 1991) and later the partial performance training like the visual perception training from Frostig (1974) or the integration training from Karma (2003).

With the beginning of school time, all exercises of reading and writing will be relevant. Mainly such practices are good to be applied as supports to the particular grades of dyslexia. Therefore, dyslexia-special classes (2nd and 3rd grade) realise a special didactic developed by Weigt (1994) with the following elements:

- Script oriented playing therapy,
- additional supporting hand signals,
- graphical signs for peculiarities of orthography, and
- a morphemic rule system for the better understanding of the construction of the German script.

These special rehabilitative classes were evaluated by Eichhorn (2017). An excellent impact on the school career and the personality development of the dyslexic children could be found.

When secondary symptoms are developed, the training methods of Betz and Breuninger (1998) can be used and shared to the children in an aggressive and an anxiety group. With both separated groups, the exercises for reducing the secondary symptoms can be applied. The exercises of reading and writing are coming later. With older individuals, these methods can be conducted also inside of psychotherapy.

# 4 Alternative New Approaches

## 4.1 Resources Oriented Intervention Approaches

The resources orientation is a new form of special education. The basic of this resources orientation is that the investigator/trainer believe that the disabled person also has other positive recourses.

All resources oriented approaches have the belief that other regions are developed and should be stimulated. For instance, those resources are virtual realities, Davis' creative learning method, reform education (e.g., free school), and Positive Psychology.

Virtual realities are used for the assessment and treatment of individuals with dyslexia by their visual-spatial strengths. Attree, Turner, and Cowell (2009) could show that the visual-spatial strengths of dyslexics are to observe in the age of adolescents not by using the traditional paper and pencil test, but computer test (e.g., British Ability Scale, BAS II), which mainly used in virtual reality tasks. The authors conclude that the learning process of dyslexic children should integrate their strengths from the beginning. In this way, they expect prevention against robust primary (failures in reading and writing) and secondary symptoms (anxiety, low self-esteem, and little motivation) of dyslexics.

In the creative learning method, Davis (2000) developed an own education by his experiences of his disorder "Dyslexia" and found out other methods, i.e., self-made plastic letters.

The reform education could show inside of the traditional, classical education (e.g., Waldorf education, Montessori education), and inside the secondary education (e.g., free school, neighbourhood school) a lot of disorder related accesses. For example, it is the Montessori material for learning the mathematical rules using "gold material".

The Positive Psychology is a field with explicit rules against the deficit orientation. In this case, a dyslexic child will be assessed for the normal side of his/her personality, and to find out the positive strengthening of his/her personality. Therefore, the assessment is not deficit-oriented.

## 4.2 Prevention Orientation

With this aim "prevention", the door to the alternative access to dyslexia is opened. Prevention can mean different things:

1. Primary prevention: Avert complete the disorder
2. Secondary prevention: Degree and generalisation of the disorder can be reduced
3. Tertiary prevention: Comorbidity or secondary symptoms can be averted

There are two examples of prevention. The first example is for children in the last year of kindergarten before they are going to school. The second example is a prevention program for parents in which the dyslexic children are not integrated.

Kuespert and Schneider (2008) developed a prevention program for children with high risk for dyslexia. It is a secondary prevention program for pre-school children with risks for dyslexia. It is a prevention program for phonological awareness for children in the last year in kindergarten.

There are some steps of the program, such as:

1. Training time: Every day with a kindergarten group with a duration of 10–15 minutes,
2. Different games in order,
3. The important impression of children "only playing",
4. Orientation on difficult children,
5. Clear articulation of the pre-school teacher, and
6. Use only phonemes not letter names.

The evaluations include three evaluation studies that give good results when the program was used in detailed. Then, after three years, there will be no long-term effects and sustainability through prediction for school achievement and prevention of school problems.

Brock and Shute (2001) developed a prevention program for parents of dyslexic children and could show very good coping results among mothers of children with dyslexia. That means a significant decrease of stress experience of mothers, more emotional binding to the child, less reported externalised behavior problems of the child and better educational competency for mothers. However, Brock and Shute could not see the changes of internalised behavior problems. This program has not yet integrated the dyslexic children. The dyslexic children are indirectly integrated only over the evaluation of the mothers.

# 5 Conclusion

This contribution wants to give an overview of the different methods of assessment and treatment currently used in the field of dyslexia. The traditional deficit orientation in assessment and treatment was added/extended by new resources and prevention-oriented approaches of assessment and intervention.

The traditional approaches which related to the theoretical hypotheses that assumed the deficit of dyslexia aim to reduce or eliminate this deficit. Therefore, the alternative new methods that attempt to find out and measure the resources or strengths of a dyslexic individual can be used as a basis for intervention and prevention.

# 6 Affiliation

Prof. Dr. Evelin Witruk
Institution: Institute of Psychology, Faculty of Life Sciences, University of Leipzig
Address: Staedtiches Kaufhaus, Neumarkt 9-19, 04109 Leipzig, Germany
E-mail: witruk@uni-leipzig.de

# 7 References

Attree, E. A., Turner, M. J., & Cowell, N. (2009). A virtual reality test identifies the visuospatial strengths of adolescents with dyslexia. *Cyberpsychological Behavior*, 12/2, 163–168.

Betz, D., & Breuninger, H. (1998). *Teufelskreis Lernstoerung*. Muenchen: PVU.

Brock, A., & Shute, R. (2001). Group Coping Skills Program for Parents of Children with Dyslexia and other Learning Disabilities. *Australian Journal of Learning Disabilities*, 6, 4, 15–25.

Davis, R. D. (2000). *Legasthenie als Talentsignal*. Muenchen: Ariston Verlag.

Dennison, P. E., & Dennison, G. (1991). *Lehrerhandbuch Brain-Gym*. Freiburg: VAK Verlag für Angewandte Kinesiologie GmbH.

Eichhorn, R. (2017). *Die Entwicklung der Sekundaersymptomatik bei Grundschulkindern mit Legasthenie in Sachsen und Sachsen-Anhalt – eine Laengsschnittuntersuchung* (Unpublished Doctoral Dissertation). University of Leipzig, Leipzig.

Frostig, M. (1974). *Visuelle Wahrnehmungsfoerderung. Uebungs- und Beobachtungsfolge für den Elementar- und Primarbereich. Anweisungsheft und Heft 1–3. (fuer deutsche Verhaeltnisse bearbeitet und herausgegeben von Anton und Erika Reinartz)*. Hannover: Schroedel.

Karma, K. (2003). *AUDILEX 2.0. Deutsche Bearbeitung von Bernd Richter*. Helsinki: Comp-Aid Ltd.

Kuespert, P., & Schneider, W. (2008). *Hoeren, Lauschen, Lernen*. Goettingen: Vandenhoeck & Ruprecht GmbH & Co. KG.

Novita, S. (2015). *Self-esteem, Anxiety, and Coping Strategies of Children with Dyslexia: A Cross-cultural Study between Indonesia and Germany* (Unpublished Doctoral Dissertation). University of Leipzig, Leipzig.

Raziq, O. (2008). *Wechselwirkungen zwischen Lese- und Rechtschreibleistung, Arbeitsge-daechtnis und Aengstlichkeit bei marokkanischen und deutschen Schuelern*. (Unpublished Doctoral Dissertation). University of Leipzig, Leipzig.

Weigt, R. (1994). *Lesen- und Schreibenlernen kann jeder!?* Methodische Hilfen bei Lese-Rechtschreib-Schwaeche. Neuwied, Kriftel, Berlin: Luchterhand.

Witruk, E. (2003). Training of working memory performance in dyslexics. *Psychology Science*, 45, I, 94–100.

Witruk, E. (2017, September). Dyslexia – does it still exist? *International Workshop of Dyslexia and Traumatic Experiences*. University of Leipzig, Leipzig.

Witruk, E., & Eichhorn, R. (2012). An Overview of Assessment and Treatment Methods of Dyslexia – with special reference to emotional and behavioral problems. *Vestnik Permskovo Univeristeta*, 2 (6), 65–76.

Mahnaz Akhavan Tafti

# Dyslexia: Disabled or Differently Abled

**Abstract:** So far, most research on dyslexia has examined the academic, behavioral and neurological deficits at the core of this syndrome. Some research, however, has looked for possible compensatory strengths associated with dyslexia. The association between dyslexia and enhancement of other functions, such as visuo-spatial abilities, creativity, differences in intellectual and cognitive development – variations known as neurodiversity – have respectively attracted much attention and widely explored. The focus of this article is on these abilities and their correlated attributes of dyslexia, such as career choice.

**Keywords:** dyslexia, visuo-spatial abilities, creativity, career choice, neurodiversity

## 1 Introduction

Dyslexia is a neurological learning disability characterized by lifelong struggles with processing the constituent sounds of words for reading and spelling in those who otherwise have the necessary intelligence, motivation and schooling (Akhavan Tafti, Boyle, & Crawford, 2014; Brunswick, Martin, & Marzano, 2010). Developmental dyslexia affects 5% - 17% of the population (Shaywitz & Shaywitz, 2005) and is typically characterized by persistent, recurrent, and universal phonological impairments (for a review of related literature, see Judge, Knox, & Caravolas, 2013); neurobiological anomalies that are related to the phonological processing that impair the episodic recall of words, dates and numbers (Pugh et al., 2000); inability for lateral masking (Geiger & Lettvin, 2000); neuroanatomical disruption in connectivity between posterior and frontal regions of the brain (Temple, 2002); deficits in visual memory and sequencing (Cortiella & Horowitz, 2014); and declarative memory deficit (Hedenius, Ullman, Alm, Jennische, & Persson, 2013; Menghini et al., 2010).

However, research, case studies, biographies, and anecdotal reports suggest that we should consider a broader range of abilities along with the known disabilities in persons with dyslexia as reflections of the differences from non-typical neurological development. Some specifically suggest that we de-stigmatize individuals with dyslexia, move away from a purely deficit perspective and emphasize the strengths that may manifest as part of the dyslexic profile. Others even suggest that individuals with dyslexia are gifted in nonverbal areas and/or that the status of being dyslexic is a gift in itself (Davis & Braun, 2010; Eide & Eide, 2012; West, 1997). The association between dyslexia and enhancement of other functions, such as visuo-spatial ability, creativity, differences in intellectual and cognitive development – variations that are regarded as neurodiversity – have respectively attracted much attention and widely explored. The focus of this chapter is on these abilities and correlated attributes of the dyslexic, such as career choices.

## 2 Visuo-spatial abilities

Developmental dyslexia were first recognized in the latter half of the 19th century, calling it 'word blindness', and it was always described as a disease of the visual system, and patients with dyslexia were frequently visited by ophthalmologists (Critchley, 1968; Shaywitz & Shaywitz, 2004). Since then, dyslexia has been linked to neuro-visual abnormalities (Bosse, Tainturier, & Valdois, 2007; Sireteanu, Goertz, Bachert, & Wandert, 2005; Skottun, 1997, 2000; Skottun & Parke, 1999; Stein, 2001; Vidyasagar & Pammer, 2010; Wright, Conlon, & Dyck, 2012) and most research has attempted to focus on the neurological deficit and its behavioral manifestations. However, substantial research has also indicated the existence of possible compensatory strengths and an association of visual-spatial talents with dyslexia (for reviews, see Akhavan Tafti et al., 2014); and similar visuo-spatial skills – neither inferior nor superior – as their average peers (see von Károlyi, Winner, Gray, & Sherman 2003; LaFrance, 1997; Martinelli & Fenech, 2017).

On the basis of anecdotal evidence, if it is to be considered, the correlation between dyslexia and superior visuo-spatial ability is robust. Several case studies have described individuals with indisputable spatial talents who may also have been dyslexic (Winner et al., 2001). Biographies of some great scientists, architects, artists, and designers have associated these individuals' reading difficulty with their superior visuo-spatial skills (West, 1997). Decades earlier, Orton (1925) had suggested that dyslexia is sometimes accompanied by spatial talents. von Károlyi (2001) found that dyslexic readers were faster, although no more accurate, in identifying impossible figures than were unimpaired readers. Witruk, Novita, Lee, & Utami (2016) confirmed the visual-spatial advantages of dyslexic individuals with regard to gender, age group and the type of orthography. A study of Polish adults with dyslexia found that mental rotation of letters was slower in these participants than in unimpaired readers although both groups were comparable when they rotated shapes (Rusiak, Lachmann, Jaskowski, & van Leeuwen, 2007).

Others have reported no differences in visuo-spatial ability between dyslexic and unimpaired readers (Brosnan, Demetre, Hamill, Robson, Shepherd, & Cody, 2002; Winner et al., 2001). Geschwind and Galaburda (1985) suggested a neurological model to explain the association between dyslexia and visual spatial talents and to account for the disproportionate incidence of individuals with dyslexia in spatial fields. They further proposed, Testosterone Hypothesis, to account for such a co-occurrence. They suggested that exposure to (or atypical sensitivity to) testosterone in utero could lead to left-hemisphere language-related deficits and resultant compensatory growth in analogous regions of the right hemisphere. This was argued to lead to brains that were symmetrical. Further empirical evidence for greater symmetry in dyslexic brains came from autopsies by Galaburda and his colleagues that showed symmetrical temporal plana in all seven of the dyslexic brains studied (Galaburda, Sherman, Rosen, Aboitiz, & Geschwind, 1985; Humphreys, Kaufmann, & Galaburda, 1990). However, the original claim was that symmetrical brains would result from inhibited left-hemisphere growth along with enhanced right-hemisphere growth. It is known that symmetrical cortical areas are associated with atypical connectivity between hemispheres (Rosen, Sherman, & Galaburda, 1989). Humphreys et al. (1990) speculated that the altered neuronal circuitry of symmetrical brains could result in varied cognitive capacities.

Some evidence from differences in visual processing of individuals with dyslexia suggest, that at least some people with dyslexia may be biased to favour information in the periphery over the centre (PCR), which accounts for the observed deficits in tasks such as visual search, but tend to exhibit peripheral advantages, as in visual comparison characteristic of a high-PCR group. Visual-spatial properties of periphery are: broad perceived field of view, high confusion from distracters or noise, high need for attention in spatial comparisons, fast processing speed, low need for working memory in spatial comparisons, good concurrent spatial processing, poor sequential visual processing, that enhance visual comparisons and implicit spatial learning (Schneps et al. as cited in Akhavan Tafti et al., 2014). Lorusso, Facoetti, Pesenti, Cattaneo, Molteni, & Geiger (2004) found that individuals with dyslexia show higher correct identification of letters in the periphery vision, supporting the notion of a different distribution of lateral masking, as a general characteristic of their visual perception, and possibly a different visual-attentional mode. Geiger & Lettvin (1987; 2000) have reported that persons with dyslexia had a markedly wider area of the peripheral field for correct identification of stimuli compared to normal readers. They found that people with dyslexia learn to read outside the foveal field and develop different strategies for tasks-directed vision.

Geiger et al. (2008) suggested that the evidence of wide visual and auditory perceptual modes in dyslexics indicates wider multi-dimensional neural tuning of sensory processing interacting with wider spatial attention. Akhavan Tafti, Hameedy, & Baghal (2009) found that students with dyslexia performed better on pictorial-spatial subtests of memory as compared to their non-dyslexic peers. Brunswick et al. (2010) have reported gender differences among men and women with and without dyslexia. They found that dyslexic men were significantly better at identifying shapes in ambiguous figures, reproducing complex figures, reproducing designs using colored blocks, and recalling the direction of the figures. They were also significantly faster and more accurate than unimpaired men at navigating and recreating a virtual environment. These data suggest that visuo-spatial advantage in dyslexia may be confined to men.

## 3 Career choice

It is important to realize that the disability in learning is often domain specific and all affected individuals may not manifest all the features detailed above. Miles (1993) suggested that dyslexic individuals show 'an unusual balance of skills'. Others refer to the dyslexic's relatively enhanced creativity and visual skills, especially in the arts or engineering sciences (Everatt, 1997). Bannatyne (1971) argued that visual spatial orientation and a preference for thinking in three dimensions in individuals with dyslexia is the reason why they gravitate to occupations which require these talents. Consistent with this view, a disproportionate incidence of individuals with reading or language weaknesses become mathematicians or major in math or science in college (Martino & Winner, 1995), inventors (Colangelo, Assouline, Kerr, Huesman, & Johnson, 1993), artists (Casey, Winner, Benbow, Hayes, & Dasilva, 1993; Steffert, 1998), and all activities that involve spatial abilities. Further, consistent with this view is the finding that late-talking children have a high proportion of relatives in spatial occupations (Sowell, 2008). Elevated numbers of people with dyslexia in careers, such as art, theatre, physics, and engineering, there is an indication of visual-spatial processing differences on neurocognitive tests; differences in brain structure; and differences in brain function for tasks not related to reading (Gilger, 2017).

Everatt, Steffert, & Smythe (1999) suggested that the coping strategies that adults with dyslexia develop to successfully overcome their difficulties may also be useful in business. Logan (2001; 2009) reported a high incidence of dyslexia among entrepreneurs. Fitzgibbon and O'Connor (2002) suggested that there is likely to be less of them in the corporate sector, as such an environment is not conducive to dyslexics (Logan, 2009). The evidence from a study on dyslexia and learning computer programming, suggests that dyslexic students bring to computer programming their visualization and creative problem-solving skills as well as their more widely recognized difficulties in spelling, organization and short-term memory (Powell, Moore, Gray, Finlay, & Reaney, 2004).

## 4 Creativity

Focusing specifically on the possible relationship between dyslexia and creativity, Everatt et al. (1999) undertook a literature review on the issue. After tracing numerous studies which investigated the relationship between creativity and dyslexia, they concluded that groups of children and adolescents with dyslexia have higher performance in tests of figural creativity than children without the disorder. Akhavan Tafti et al. (2009) found that students with dyslexia showed superiority – though not significant – on the fluency and flexibility subtests of creativity. Studies undertaken by Corlu, Ozcan, & Korkmazlar (2007; 2009) observed better creative performance in children with dyslexia. The authors compared drawings produced by two groups of individuals with and without dyslexia. Greater richness of details and greater speed in producing the pictures was observed in the drawings of the subjects with dyslexia (Alves & Nakano, 2014).

While in other research, Łockiewicz, Bogdanowicz, & Bogdanowicz, (2014) found similar creative performance in children with and without dyslexia. Wolff & Lundberg (2002) have noted that art academy students reported significantly more signs of dyslexia than non-art university students. People with dyslexia often have a natural flair for one or more of the arts such as music, dance, drawing or acting. They also often possess a natural ability to see patterns in noise, producing creative abstract ideas out of what many would look upon as ordinary sensory environments (Chakravarty, 2009). Critchley (1968) and Miller (2008) postulated that the inferior parietal lobule, especially in the non-dominant hemisphere is the seat of visuo-spatial cognition, mathematical ideation and imagery movement as also of artistic and literal creativity. It is supposed that normally the dominant hemisphere has an inhibitory influence on creative functions on the non-dominant parietal lobe. Some case histories support the notion that a dominant hemispheric dysfunction may lead to 'dis-inhibited' functioning of the non-dominant parietal lobe to result in the unmasking of hidden artistic talent. A phenomenon identified much earlier by Kapur (1996) which he called 'paradoxical functional facilitation', which is a compensatory enhancement occurring as a specific manifestation of central nervous system (CNS) plasticity (Chakravarty, 2009).

In extensive research, LaFrance (1997) compared three groups of gifted, gifted-dyslexic, and dyslexic age-matched students on cognitive and creative thinking differences. Results showed that gifted/dyslexic students exhibited strength in expressing humour, problem solving, capturing the essence of an idea, synthesising dissimilar concepts, expressed feelings of being in control in their writing, expressed feelings better in form completion than in words, and positive and negative feelings in their drawings. Like dyslexics, gifted/dyslexics expressed intuitive aspects of creative thinking but were somewhat stronger in gaining information through their physical senses. Also, gifted/dyslexic students were stronger than the gifted in synthesising incomplete figures. Originality was not a discriminating factor because it was equal in students who were dyslexic, gifted and gifted/dyslexic. In scenario writing, the dyslexic children were almost as strong as those who were gifted in expressing positive and negative feelings toward themselves and the future. The students who were dyslexic scored higher than the two gifted groups on the resistance to premature closure, an intuitive creative aspect. On the creative strengths, dyslexic students scored higher than the two gifted groups in Fantasy, were similar to the gifted in unusual visualization, and equal to both gifted groups in extending boundaries. In all cognitive and physical sensing aspects of creative thinking, the gifted group was the strongest.

## 5 Neurodiversity

Neurodiversity – a portmanteau of neurological and diversity – is an approach to learning and disability that advocates that diverse neurological conditions are the result of normal variations in the human genome. Neurodiversity is a concept where atypical neurological development and variations are to be recognized and respected as any other human differences. As a challenge to the prevailing pathological views of neurological diversity with attached social stigmas, this approach frames autistic spectrum, attention deficit hyperactivity disorder/attention deficit disorder (ADHD/ADD), dyslexia, dyspraxia, dyscalculia, and other neurotypes as a natural human variation that should be accepted and valued as a social category like gender, ethnicity, and sexual orientation (Hendrickx, 2010; Jaarsma & Welin, 2012). He instead proposed the term "neurominority" as a good, non-pathologizing word for referring to all people who are not neurotypical. Walker (2012) believes that people with other neurological styles are poorly accommodated and marginalized by the dominant culture. Blume (1998) did not use the term neurodiversity, but instead, he described the foundation of the idea in the phrase "neurological pluralism". In compensation models of dyslexia, the specific-talent hypothesis can stand alone but fits well as a subordinate category of neurodiversity.

Geshwind (1982) termed the association of a deficit with talent as the pathology of superiority and suggested that people with dyslexia excel in domains such as architecture, art, and engineering (Tobias, 2004). Proponents of neurodiversity, advocate promotion of support systems like inclusion-focused educational and social services and accommodations, occupational training, communication and assistive technologies, and independent living support, to allow those who are *non-neurotypical* to live their lives, as they believe them to be authentic forms of human diversity, self-expression, and being. Acquiring a 'difference' view about themselves is very important for the well-being and coherency of neurodiversity people. In their research, Griffin & Pollak (2009) separated 27 students (with autism, dyslexia, developmental coordination disorder, ADHD, and stroke) into two categories of self-view: a 'difference' view or a 'medical/deficit' view. They found that although all of the students reported uniformly difficult schooling careers involving exclusion, abuse, and bullying. Those who viewed themselves from a difference view (41%) indicated higher academic self-esteem and confidence in their abilities, and many (73%) expressed considerable career ambitions with positive and clear goals. Neurological evidence is consistent with the possibility that dyslexic brains are atypical in the structure, development, and organization of their cells and might process visual-spatial information in an atypical manner (Galaburda et al., 1985; Humphreys et al., 1990); as well as at the gross anatomical level; dyslexic brains are also atypical in patterns of hemispheric activation during both linguistic and non-linguistic tasks (Helenius, Salmelin, Service, & Connolly, 1999; Rumsey, 1996; Shaywitz & Shaywitz as cited in von Károlyi et al., 2003).

Few empirical studies (e.g., Olulade et al., 2012; Diehl et al. as cited in Gilger, 2017) have reported differences in the neurological functioning of persons with dyslexia. These studies of complex visual-spatial reasoning suggest that while dyslexics perform spatial reasoning problems, their functional neurology is different from that of normally reading peers; even if their outward test performance is at or below that of normal readers. That is, the underlying brain processes may differ even when observed behaviors do not. A Hong Kong study, using fMRI technology, has recently shown that the children are reading English – an alphabetic language – used a different part of the brain than those reading Chinese – a non-alphabetic language (Chakravarty, 2009).

For Armstrong (2010), the nature of neurodiversity can be described through the concept of multiple intelligences (MI). He asserts that one of the major reasons that people with intellectual differences have had a problem integrating into the mainstream of society is that they fail to comply with a single innate and fixed entity measurement. He proposes, once we comprehend Gardner's MI theory, especially its neurological component, it becomes easier to understand the reason for the different cognitive profiles of neurodiverse individuals. We can see, e.g. the verbal and linguistic deficits of dyslexics, as well as their visuo-spatial talents and interpersonal gifts. LaFrance (1997) emphasized on Gardner's notion that special educators have long known that individuals learn differently and that education is most effective when these individual differences are recognized and addressed. He also noted that children who are dyslexic often show enhanced facility at visual and/or spatial tasks. In the study of Akhavan Tafti, Heidarzadeh, & Khademi (2014), they compared MI profile of students with and without learning disabilities (LD). Results showed no significant difference in Musical, Bodily/Kinesthetic, Intrapersonal, and Natural Intelligence scores in two groups. However, it is significantly higher on Linguistic, Logical/ Mathematical, and Interpersonal Intelligence scores in students without LD; and significantly higher Spatial Intelligence scores in LD students. The *acceptance perspective* recommended by this approach is a view that *non-neurotypicals* such as autism, learning disabilities and the like are not disorders, but normal incidents of alternate variation in brain wiring or a less common expression of the human genome. Proponents of this perspective believe that these are a unique way of being and their uniqueness should be validated, and supported as the differences of any other minority group should be tolerated rather than avoided, discriminated against or eliminated (Gal, 2007; Waltz, as cited in Akhavan Tafti, 2017).

# 6 Discussion

It is clear that people with dyslexia have relative strengths or profiles of cognitive abilities, where some skills are relatively low, and others are relatively high. Investigating the strengths of dyslexia is a new area of research, which requires providing operational definitions for strengths, developing standardized assessments, and conducting empirical studies. The development of above-average compensatory skills in a specific area, such as the visual-spatial domain, and the empirical documentation that dyslexia co-occurred with greater-than-average visual-spatial abilities in a high proportion of affected individuals, would be highly useful information. It is a scientific and social responsibility to determine to what extent the assertions of special talents in dyslexics can be supported, and then to identify how best to tailor clinical and educational interventions to help students make the best of the abilities they possess, and in guiding dyslexics in their career choices. It would be beneficial to allow children with dyslexia to develop their unique artistic ability or other talents to its full capacity and not to over-emphasize the remedial training for the correction of the disturbed symbol coding operations.

Although findings suggest that dyslexic differences likely encompass more than reading-related problems but, this question is still relevant: is there sufficient scientific evidence to support this notion? There are some unanswered questions regarding the underlying neurology and behavioral expression of the dyslexic brain as it pertains to the domains of reasoning, creativity, and the processing of non-linguistic/nonverbal information, we need more well-designed research examining these issues. Given the complex and multifaceted nature of visual functioning, it is unlikely that any single factor alone (including all the factors discussed here) can account for all of the rich variability inherent in the dyslexic phenotype. Additional research is required to examine the visual differences and possible strengths further.

Reasons for the inconsistencies in results may be due to different methodologies, heterogeneous samples and small samples. Moreover, there may be no genuine spatial superiority in dyslexia and the findings reported may be artefacts arising from speculations about famous dyslexic individuals, well-known exemplars are persuasive, but they may not be representative. Many historical studies are unreliable because there is no way of properly assessing reading difficulties in the past great scientists and artists, and more importantly, there is the danger of finding what one is looking for. These great names may be dyslexic, but there are substantially more who are not. Winner et al. (2001) and von Kàrolyi et al. (2003) suggested that there is a need for greater ecological validity, as the studies employing artificial visuo-spatial tasks may not reveal superior performance by dyslexic participants because such skills would only be salient in authentic tasks that are practical in nature.

## 7 Affiliation

Dr. Mahnaz Akhavan Tafti
Institution: Alzahra University
Address: College of Education & Psychology, Alzahra University, Vanak, Tehran, Iran, Postal Code: 1993893973.
E-mail: makhavan@alzahra.ac.ir

## 8 References

Akhavan Tafti, M. (2017). *A new look to the old problems of learning disorders.* Tehran, Iran: Tehran Iranian Students Book Agency Publication.

Akhavan Tafti, M., Boyle, J. R., & Crawford, C. M. (2014). Meta-analysis of visual-spatial deficits in dyslexia. *International Journal of Brain and Cognitive Sciences, 3*(1), 25–34. doi:10.5923/j.ijbcs.20140301.03

Akhavan Tafti, M., Hameedy, M. A., & Baghal, N. M. (2009). Dyslexia, a deficit or a difference: Comparing the creativity and memory skills of dyslexic and nondyslexic students in Iran. *Social Behavior and Personality: An International Journal, 37*(8), 1009–1016. doi:10.2224/sbp.2009.37.8.1009

Akhavan Tafti, M., Heidarzadeh, M., & Khademi, M. (2014). A comparison of Multiple Intelligences profile of students with and without learning disabilities. *International Journal of Applied Psychology, 4*(3), 121–125. doi:10.5923/j.ijap.20140403.06

Alves, R. J. R., & Nakano, T. D. C. (2014). Creativity and intelligence in children with and without developmental dyslexia1. *Paidéia (Ribeirão Preto), 24*(59), 361–369.

Armstrong, T. (2010). *Neurodiversity: Discovering the extraordinary gifts of autism, ADHD, dyslexia, and other brain differences.* Lebanon: Da Capo Press.

Bannatyne, A. (1971). *Language, reading, and learning disabilities: Psychology, neuropsychology, diagnosis and remediation.* Springfield, IL: Charles C. Thomas Publisher.

Bascom, J. (2012). *Loud hands: Autistic people, speaking.* Washington, DC: Autism Self-Advocacy Network Press.

Blume, H. (1998). Neurodiversity. *Atlantic, 30.*

Bosse, M. L., Tainturier, M. J., & Valdois, S. (2007). Developmental dyslexia: The visual attention span deficit hypothesis. *Cognition, 104*(2), 198–230.

Brosnan, M., Demetre, J., Hamill, S., Robson, K., Shepherd, H., & Cody, G. (2002). Executive functioning in adults and children with developmental dyslexia. *Neuropsychologia, 40*(12), 2144–2155. doi:10.1016/S0028-3932(02)00046-5

Brunswick, N., Martin, G. N., & Marzano, L. (2010). Visuospatial superiority in developmental dyslexia: Myth or reality? *Learning and Individual Differences, 20*(5), 421–426. doi:10.1016/j.lindif.2010.04.007

Casey, M. B., Winner, E., Benbow, C., Hayes, R., & Dasilva, D. (1993). Skill at image generation: Handedness interacts with strategy preference for individuals majoring in spatial fields. *Cognitive Neuropsychology, 10*(1), 57–77.

Chakravarty, A. (2009). Artistic talent in dyslexia—A hypothesis. *Medical Hypotheses, 73*(4), 569–571. doi:10.1016/j.mehy.2009.05.034

Colangelo, N., Assouline, S. G., Kerr, B., Huesman, R., & Johnson, D. (1993). *Mechanical inventiveness: A three-phase study.* In Ciba Foundation, *Ciba Foundation Symposium, 178. The origins and development of high ability* (pp. 160–174). Oxford, England: John Wiley & Sons. doi:10.1002/9780470514498.ch10

Corlu, M., Ozcan, O., & Korkmazlar, U. (2007). The potential of dyslexic individuals in communication design education. *Behavioural Neurology, 18*(4), 217–223.

Corlu, M., Ozcan, O., & Korkmazlar, U. (2009). The meaning of dyslexics' drawings in communication design. *Dyslexia, 15*(2), 148–154. doi:10.1002/dys.362

Cortiella, C., & Horowitz, S. H. (2014). *The state of learning disabilities: Facts, trends and emerging issues.* New York: National Center for Learning Disabilities.

Critchley, M. (1968). Developmental dyslexia. *Pediatric Clinics of North America, 15*(3), 669–676. doi:10.1016/S0031-3955(16)32168-X

Davis, R. D., & Braun, E. M. (2010). *The gift of dyslexia*. New York: Penguin Group.

Eide, B. L., & Eide, F. F. (2012). *The dyslexic advantage: Unlocking the hidden potential of the dyslexic brain*. New York: Penguin Group.

Everatt, J. (1997). The abilities and disabilities associated with adult developmental dyslexia. *Journal of Research in Reading, 20*(1), 13–21. doi:10.1111/1467-9817.00016

Everatt, J., Steffert, B., & Smythe, I. (1999). An eye for the unusual: Creative thinking in dyslexics. *Dyslexia, 5*(1), 28–46.

Galaburda, A. M., Sherman, G. F., Rosen, G. D., Aboitiz, F., & Geschwind, N. (1985). Developmental dyslexia: four consecutive patients with cortical anomalies. *Annals of Neurology, 18*(2), 222–233. doi:10.1002/ana.410180210

Geiger, G., & Lettvin, J. Y. (1987). Peripheral vision in persons with dyslexia. *The New England Journal of Medicine, 316*(20), 1238–1243.

Geiger, G., & Lettvin, J. Y. (2000). Developmental dyslexia: A different perceptual strategy and how to learn a new strategy for reading. *Saggi CD and D, 26*, 73–89.

Geiger, G., Cattaneo, C., Galli, R., Pozzoli, U., Lorusso, M. L., Facoetti, A., Pozzoli, U., Lorusso, M. L., Facoetti, A., & Molteni, M. (2008). Wide and diffuse perceptual modes characterize dyslexics in vision and audition. *Perception, 37*(11), 1745–1764. doi:10.1068/p6036

Geschwind, N., & Galaburda, A. M. (1985). Cerebral lateralization: Biological Mechanisms, Associations, and Pathology: A Hypothesis and a Program for Research. *Archives of Neurology, 42*(5):428–459. doi:10.1001/archneur.1985.04060050026008

Gilger, J. W. (2017). Beyond a reading disability: comments on the need to examine the full spectrum of abilities/disabilities of the atypical dyslexic brain. *Annals of Dyslexia, 67*(2), 1–5. doi:10.1007/s11881-017-0142-x

Griffin, E., & Pollak, D. (2009). Student experiences of neurodiversity in higher education: insights from the BRAINHE project. *Dyslexia, 15*(1), 23–41. doi:10.1002/dys.383

Hedenius, M., Ullman, M. T., Alm, P., Jennische, M., & Persson, J. (2013). Enhanced recognition memory after incidental encoding in children with developmental dyslexia. *PloS one, 8*(5), e63998. doi:10.1371/journal.pone.0063998

Hendrickx, S. (2010). *The adolescent and adult neuro-diversity handbook: Asperger's syndrome, ADHD, dyslexia, dyspraxia, and related conditions*. Philadelphia: Jessica Kingsley Publishers.

Humphreys, P., Kaufmann, W. E., & Galaburda, A. M. (1990). Developmental dyslexia in women: Neuropathological findings in three patients. *Annals of Neurology, 28*(6), 727–738. doi:10.1002/ana.410280602

Jaarsma, P., & Welin, S. (2012). Autism as a natural human variation: Reflections on the claims of the neurodiversity movement. *Health Care Analysis, 20*(1), 20–30.

Judge, J., Knox, P. C., & Caravolas, M. (2013). Spatial orienting of attention in dyslexic adults using directional and alphabetic cues. *Dyslexia, 19*(2), 55–75.

LaFrance, E. D. B. (1997). The gifted/dyslexic child: Characterizing and addressing strengths and weaknesses. *Annals of Dyslexia, 47*(1), 163–182. doi:10.1007/s11881-997-0025-7

Łockiewicz, M., Bogdanowicz, K. M., Bogdanowicz, M. (2014). Psychological resources of adults with developmental dyslexia. *Journal of Learning Disabilities, 47*(6), 543–555.

Logan, J. (2009). Dyslexic entrepreneurs: The incidence; their coping strategies and their business skills. *Dyslexia, 15*(4), 328–346. doi:10.1002/dys.388

Logan, J. M. (2001). *Entrepreneurial success: A study of the incidence of dyslexia in the entrepreneurial population and the influence of dyslexia upon the entrepreneur.* Bristol: University of Bristol.

Lorusso, M., Facoetti, A., Pesenti, S., Cattaneo, C., Molteni, M., & Geiger, G. (2004). Wider recognition in peripheral vision common to different subtypes of dyslexia. *Vision research, 44*(20), 2413–2424. doi:10.1016/j.visres.2004.05.001

Martinelli, V., & Fenech, D. (2017). Dyslexia and Enhanced Visuospatial Ability: A Maltese Study. *Academic Journal of Interdisciplinary Studies, 6*(1), 103.

Martino, G., & Winner, E. (1995). Talents and disorders-relationships among handedness, sex, and college major. *Brain and Cognition, 29*(1), 66–84.

Menghini, D., Finzi, A., Benassi, M., Bolzani, R., Facoetti, A., Giovagnoli, S., Vicari, S. (2010). Different underlying neurocognitive deficits in developmental dyslexia: A comparative study. *Neuropsychologia, 48*(4), 863–872.

Miles, T. (1993). *Dyslexia: The pattern of difficulties.* London: Whurr Publishers.

Miller, B. L. (2008). Creativity in the context of neurologic illness. *CNS Spectrums, 13*(S2), 7–9. doi:10.1017/S1092852900002820

Orton, S. T. (1925). "Word-Blindness" in School Children. *Archives of Neurology and Psychiatry, 14*(5). doi:10.1001/archneurpsyc.1925.02200170002001

Powell, N., Moore, D., Gray, J., Finlay, J., & Reaney, J. (2004). *Dyslexia and learning computer programming.* London: Taylor & Francis.

Pugh, K. R., Mencl, W. E., Shaywitz, B. A., Shaywitz, S. E., Fulbright, R. K., Constable, R. T., Gore, J. C. (2000). The angular gyrus in developmental dyslexia: Task-specific differences in functional connectivity within posterior cortex. *Psychological Science, 11*(1), 51–56.

Rosen, G., Sherman, G., & Galaburda, A. (1989). Interhemispheric connections differ between symmetrical and asymmetrical brain regions. *Neuroscience, 33*(3), 525–533.

Rusiak, P., Lachmann, T., Jaskowski, P., & van Leeuwen, C. (2007). Mental rotation of letters and shapes in developmental dyslexia. *Perception*, *36*(4), 617–631. doi:10.1068/p5644

Shaywitz, S. E., & Shaywitz, B. A. (2004). Reading disability and the brain. *Educational Leadership*, 61(6), 6–11.

Shaywitz, S. E., & Shaywitz, B. A. (2005). Dyslexia (specific reading disability). *Biological Psychiatry*, *57*(11), 1301–1309. doi:10.1016/j.biopsych.2005.01.043

Sireteanu, R., Goertz, R., Bachert, I., & Wandert, T. (2005). Children with developmental dyslexia show a left visual "minineglect". *Vision research*, *45*(25), 3075–3082.

Skottun, B. C. (1997). Some remarks on the magnocellular deficit theory of dyslexia. *Vision Research*, *37*(7), 965–966.

Skottun, B. C. (2000). The magnocellular deficit theory of dyslexia: The evidence from contrast sensitivity. *Vision Research*, *40*(1), 111–127.

Skottun, B. C., & Parke, L. A. (1999). The possible relationship between visual deficits and dyslexia: examination of a critical assumption. *Journal of Learning Disabilities*, *32*(1), 2–5. doi:10.1177/002221949903200101

Sowell, T. (2008). *Late-talking children*. Cambridge, MA: The MIT Press.

Steffert, B. (1998). Sign minds and design minds. *Creative thinking: Towards broader horizons*. Malta: Malta University Press.

Stein, J. (2001). The magnocellular theory of developmental dyslexia. *Dyslexia*, *7*(1), 12–36.

Temple, E. (2002). Brain mechanisms in normal and dyslexic readers. *Current Opinion in Neurobiology*, *12*(2), 178–183. doi:10.1016/S0959-4388(02)00303-3

Tobias, H. D. (2004). *Focus on Dyslexia Research*. New York: Nova Publishers.

Vidyasagar, T. R., & Pammer, K. (2010). Dyslexia: A deficit in visuo-spatial attention, not in phonological processing. *Trends in Cognitive Sciences*, *14*(2), 57–63.

Votalent: Global visual-spatial ability. *Brain and Language*, *85*(3), 427–431.

Walker, N. (2012). In J. Bascom (Ed.), *Loud Hands: Autistic People, Speaking*, 154–162. Washington, DC: The Autistic Press.

West, T. G. (1997). Slow words, quick images–dyslexia as an advantage in tomorrow's workplace. *Learning Disabilities and Employment*, 349–370.

Winner, E., von Káarolyi, C., Malinsky, D., French, L., Seliger, C., Ross, E., & Weber, C. (2001). Dyslexia and visual-spatial talents: Compensation vs deficit model. *Brain and Language*, *76*(2), 81–110. doi:10.1006/brln.2000.2392

Witruk, E., Novita, S., Lee, Y., & Utami, D. S. (Eds). (2016). *Dyslexia and Traumatic Experiences* (Vol. 7). Frankfurt am Main, Germany: Peter Lang. GmbH.

Wolff, U., & Lundberg, I. (2002). The prevalence of dyslexia among art students. *Dyslexia, 8*(1), 34–42. doi:10.1002/dys.211

Wright, C. M., Conlon, E. G., & Dyck, M. (2012). Visual search deficits are independent of magnocellular deficits in dyslexia. *Annals of Dyslexia, 62*(1), 53–69.

Samudra Senarath

# Anxiety and Self-Esteem among Children with Dyslexia in Sri Lanka

**Abstract:** Dyslexia is a complex neurological condition, occurring in approximately five to twelve percent of the population. For more than a decade, the impacts of secondary symptoms on the lives of individuals with dyslexia have been studied from different perspectives. The present study was focused to identify children with dyslexia anxiety and the level of their self-esteem as well as confidence in education compared to the non-dyslexia children. A total of 30 children with and without dyslexia, living in the Western Province participated in this study. These children, studying in Grade five in boy's schools, belonged to the age group of 10–11 years. All these children were given three questionnaires (i.e., Spence Children's Anxiety Scale, Culture-Free Self-Esteem Inventories 3). Self-developed screen test and semi-structured interviews were also conducted to examine the confidence in education. Descriptive analysis, paired sample t-test, and frequency analysis were used to test hypotheses. Results of this study showed that the children with dyslexia have not displayed a significant level of overall anxiety scores. Compared to the anxiety subscales; Generalized, Separation, and Social anxiety, and some items presented significant differences in children with dyslexia in contrast to the normal children. Children with dyslexia have shown significantly very low self-esteem in contrast to the normal children. It is identified that normal children also showed the self-esteem below the average level. Very low level of confidence in education is noticed in the group of children with dyslexia when compared to the normal children.

**Keywords:** children with dyslexia, anxiety, self-esteem, confidence in education

## 1 Problem of the Study

Research on dyslexia states that some children have great difficulty in learning to read, write, spell and pronounce the words, despite having normal intelligence. The prevailing rate of dyslexia is 5% - 12% in the present world (Katusic, Colligan, Barbaresi, Schaid, & Jacobsaon, 2001). However, Sri Lankan literature reports the prevailing rate is 5–10%. Researchers have stated that the primary symptoms of dyslexia in early school children are poor identification and knowledge of sounds, low awareness of phoneme and problems with coping. Because of dyslexia, many children are dropped from the schools (Bolhasan, 2009). It has long been hypothesised that children with learning disabilities, including dyslexia, may be highly vulnerable to emotional consequences such as anxiety, stress, somatic complaints etc. One of the research study proved that 20% of children with dyslexia suffer from depression and another 20% suffer from anxiety disorders. Studies show that the most dyslexia pre-schoolers do not suffer from anxiety, but their anxiety develops as they enter into school and experience difficulties to fit the learning environment and expectations of teachers and parents (Bolhasan, 2009).

In general, children with learning difficulties reported that a low score of positive well-being, were unhappy and more anxious than their peers (Casey, Levy, Brown, & Brooks-Gunn, 1992). Children with dyslexia have more academic, social and psychological problems than their non-dyslexia peers (Vigilante & Dane, 1991). Many researchers stated that appropriate teaching and support could help to make a progress in children with dyslexia and decrease their secondary psychological symptoms. In Sri Lankan context, this area is novel to teachers and officers in education system. As a result of this, teachers have less knowledge, misconceptions, and low experiences. Inadequate teacher training programmes, lack of time for contact, being overloaded with daily school routines and responsibilities prevent helping these children (Senarath, 2016). In Sri Lanka, education system mainly focuses on three competitive national exams, e.g., the Grade-Five Scholarship Examination, the General Examination of Ordinary Level and the General Examination of Advanced Level. There are lacks of sufficient studies on secondary symptoms of children with dyslexia. The primary objective of the present study is to identify the anxiety level among children with dyslexia in contrast to the non-dyslexia children. The study expects to examine the level of self-esteem among children with dyslexia and the confidence shows in education during the learning period in the regular classroom. Specific hypotheses were made for each goal of this study. Thus, dyslexia children would have significantly higher anxieties, low self-esteem and low confidence in education in comparison to the normal children.

## 2 Theoretical Review

Scientific research on dyslexia has been increased over the past several decades. Nevertheless, numbers of existing studies are carried out to investigate the nature, aetiology, and assessment methods. On the research studies in secondary psychological symptoms of anxiety, depression, self-confidence, self-esteem and motivation are limited. According to the research evidence children and adolescents with dyslexia have higher anxiety levels than typically developing children. For instance, Paget's and Reynold's (1984) study found that those with 6 to 17-year-old children with learning disabilities were more anxious than their non-learning disabled peers, as the anxiety manifesting itself to worry and concentration difficulties.

Further, Casey, Levy, Brown, and Brooks-Gunn (1992) conducted a study and reported that children (aged 8–12 years) with reading and writing difficulties displayed significantly lower scores for positive well-being, and were unhappier and anxious than their peers who have no difficulty in reading. In a review of research on children population with learning difficulties, Huntington and Bender (1993) concluded that children with learning difficulties might experience higher levels of anxiety than their peers. Willcutt and Pennington (2000) examined the psychiatric difficulties present in a sample of reading disabled twins. They found that anxiety was associated with reading difficulties, but, in contrast hyperactivity and conduct disorder were not elevated in twins among reading disabled children. This suggests that increased anxiety levels occur as a consequence of language difficulties, rather than being caused by the genetic and environmental influences common to both twins. Based on the findings of the above discussions, it is expected that children with dyslexia will show more trait anxiety regarding academic situations than controls. Eichhorn (2016) study proved that children with in integrative classes showed a lack of scholastic self-esteem significantly when compared with the control group.

# 3 Methods

## 3.1 Sample

The sample survey design and random sampling techniques were selected for this study. Fifteen children with dyslexia and fifteen normal children were selected in grade five classes (age 10–11 years) from three schools in educational zone, Colombo.

## 3.2 Instrument

Two Standardized tests were employed for the present study. These are the Spence Children Anxiety Scale (SCAS) (Spence, 1998). Test reliability and validity presented ($\alpha$ = 0.71) and ($r$ = .58) three editions of Culture-Free Self-Esteem Inventories (CFSEI-3) (Battle, 2002). For the current study reliability and validity are stated as ($\alpha$ = 0.78). Self-developed screening questionnaire reliability and validity showed ($\alpha$ = 0.67). Semi-structured interviews were also conducted with ten students in both the groups. Quantitative data analyzes were used for children's anxiety, and self-esteem which measures mean, and standard deviation and paired t-test. Confidence in education was analyzed by using percentages. Semi-structured interviews were presented as descriptive as well as percentage vice.

# 4 Results of the Study

Children with dyslexia and normal children did not present significantly for the overall anxiety scores. But in contrast, the generalised anxiety subscale presented anxiety children with dyslexia (Experimental Group, EG) compared to the normal children (Control Group, CG) as mentioned in Figure 1. Children with dyslexia presented generalised anxiety symptoms five out of six items, were proved their anxiety in contrast to the normal children; "I feel worry about things" (EG $M$ = 3.08, $SD$ = 0.76), CG ($M$ = 1.76, $SD$ = 0.70), $p$ < 0.001; "When I have problem, my heart beats really fast" (EG; $M$ = 3.07, $SD$ = 0.78); (CG $M$ = 1.74, $SD$ = 0.74), $p$ < 0.001.)"

## Generalized Anxiety

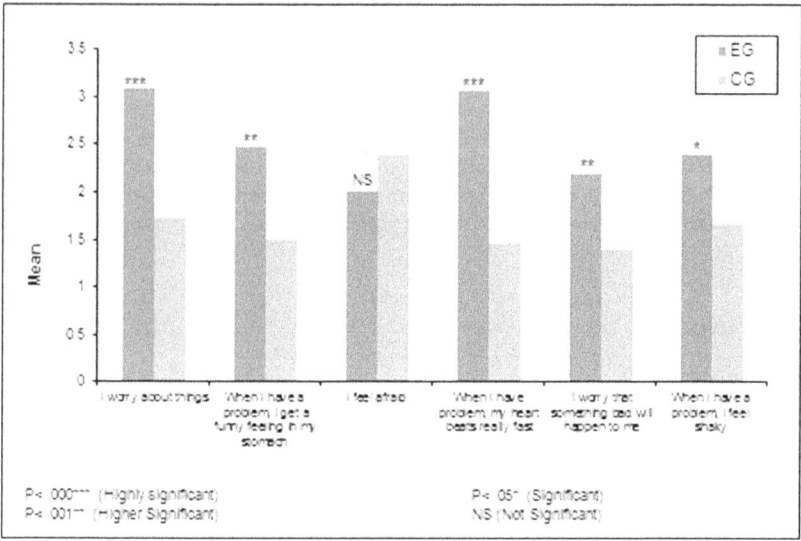

Figure 1. Generalised anxiety in two groups

Results of semi-structured interviews are also proved that children with dyslexia have more worries about their classroom performances. Children often experience actual physical symptoms due to their anxiety, and this is turned to decrease in their ability to learn or to be absent from the school. And interview results verified that children with dyslexia presented other difficulties such as fatigue, irritability, headaches, distress, misbehavior to avoid a task, lack of participation in class discussions or activities, negative talk about self, easily frustrated, reluctant to ask for help, expressing anger, etc.

According to the Table 1, children with dyslexia encountered social anxiety significantly in comparison to the normal children. (i.e., "I feel scared when I have to take test" (EG; $M = 3.33$, $SD = 0.82$); (CG; $M = 1.27$, $SD = 0.59$); $p < 0.001$; "I worry that I will do badly at my school work" (EG; $M = 3.00$, $SD = 1.07$); (CG; $M = 1.60$, $SD = 0.83$), $p < 0.001$; "I feel afraid if I have to talk in front of my class" ($M = 3.07$, $SD = 1.03$); (CG; $M = 1.03$, $SD = 0.26$), $p < 0.001$). Interview results were also revealed that children with dyslexia were unable to cope up with the difficulties within educational activities in the classroom with compared to the normal children. Term test marks of children with dyslexia are very low and classroom rank was also back behind the all normal children.

**Table 1.** Social anxiety in both groups

| Social anxiety | Mean | | SD | | Significant |
|---|---|---|---|---|---|
| | Experimental Group | Control Group | Experimental Group | Control Group | |
| I feel scared when I have to take test | 3.33 | 1.27 | 0.82 | 0.59 | 0.000*** |
| I feel afraid if I have to use public toilets or bathrooms | 2.47 | 1.33 | 1.13 | 0.82 | 0.004** |
| I feel afraid that I will make a fool of myself in front of people | 3.00 | 2.47 | 1.07 | 1.19 | 0.207 |
| I worry that I will do badly at my school work | 3.00 | 1.60 | 1.07 | 0.83 | 0.000*** |
| I worry that other people think of me | 3.00 | 1.20 | 1.00 | 0.41 | 0.000*** |
| I feel afraid if I have to talk in front of my class | 3.07 | 1.07 | 1.03 | 0.26 | 0.000*** |

Note. $p < 0.001$***, $p < 0.01$**, $p < 0.05$*. SD: Standard Deviation

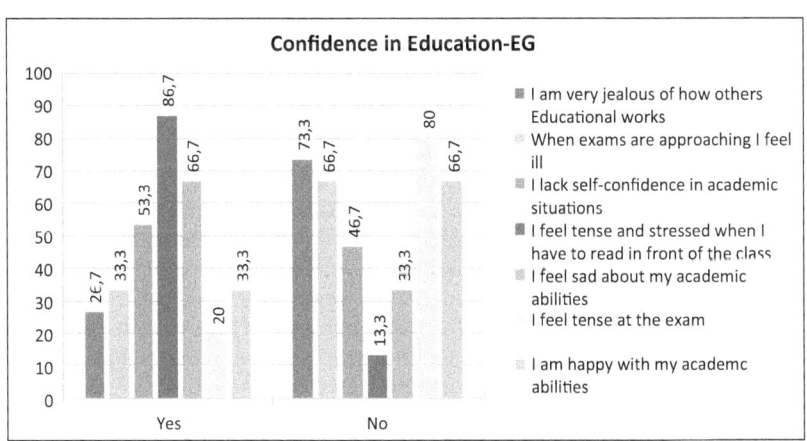

**Figure 2.** Confidence in Education - Experimental Group (Children with Dyslexia)

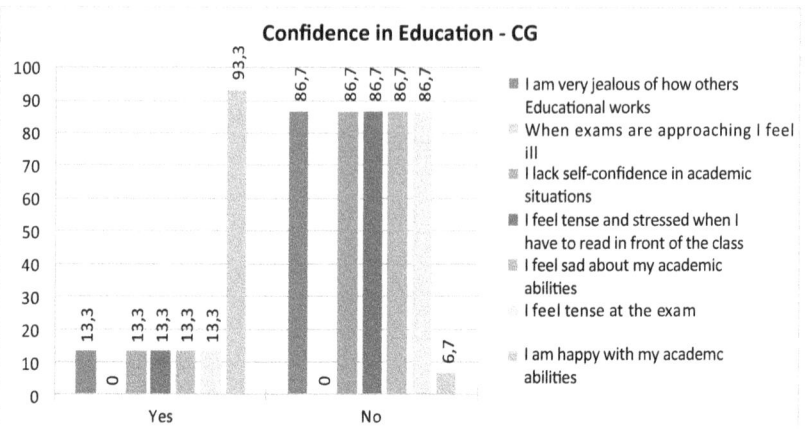

**Figure 3.** Confidence in Education – Control Group (Normal Children)

According to the third objective of the study, the findings of the research proved that children with dyslexia faced significant difficulties in education in contrast to the normal children. According to figure 2, experimental group of children encountered worries, sadness about their abilities in education, tense at the exam and feel ill significantly in compared to the figure 3, in non-dyslexia children. Lack of self-confidence in academic situations presented higher level in EG in contrast to CG, i.e., "yes response" was in EG = 53.3% and CG presented 13.3%, but no responses were reported in CG 86.7%. Accordingly, the results of interview also proved children with dyslexia and their parents are frustrated about the educational level of their children. Children with dyslexia complained that they cannot do the work assign to them throughout the day, but their peers learned quickly. Children with dyslexia often expressed the feelings of embarrassment, humiliation, anxiety, anger, frustration and guilt. According to the figure 2, children with dyslexia, often were tensed and stressed when they have to read in front of the class. It was presented as 86.7%; sad about academic abilities 66.7% and "I am happy with my academic abilities" was 33.3% in contrast to the non-dyslexia children respectively.

By administering the CFSEI-3 scale for both the groups, findings showed that children with dyslexia presented a low level of self-esteem quotient (GSEQ < 70) in contrast to the normal children, but normal children are also presented below average quotient (GSEQ = 80–89). The GSEQ's from 90–110 is considered normal quotient. Compared to the findings, children with dyslexia showed significant anxieties and difficulties in classroom activities. In contrast, both the groups of the children had to sit the grade five national exam within three months. Accordingly, these difficulties influenced to decrease the self-esteem of the children in both the groups.

Table 2. Level of Self Esteem between EG & CG

| Group | Mean | SD | Global Self Esteem Quotients (GSEQ) |
|---|---|---|---|
| EG (Dyslexic) | 49 | 10.67 | < 70 Very low self esteem |
| CG (Non-dyslexic) | 82 | 8.32 | 80 – 89 Below average self esteem |

## 5 Discussion, Conclusion and Suggestions

Chidlren with dyslexia presented a certain level of anxieties within subscales and low level of self-esteem in compared to normal children. However, the CG group performed below the average level of self-esteem statistically. This was also verified with interview results, such as the CG group chidlren were also faced Grade-Five National Exam which also influenced the decrease of their self-esteem. They are always frustrated and faced with difficulties every day at school. Experimental group of children presented the higher level of educational problems than non-dyslexia children. According to the findings, hypotheses were accepted that means children with dyslexia were showed very low self-esteem and difficulty with confidence in education in compared to the normal children.

Based on the findings of this research study, dyslexia children have shown the generalised and social anxieties, education difficulties, and very low self-esteem quotient in contrast to the non-dyslexia children. Teachers need more training on dyslexia children more teaching facilities, and teaching-learning aids; improve remedial teaching methods especially for chidlren with dyslexia; need proper counselling service for children with dyslexia and their parents. The examination procedure is needed to be changed to measure the academic performance among children with dyslexia, and that would be supportive of preventing psychological issues.

## 6 Affiliation

Dr. Samudra Senarath
Institution: University of Colombo, Department of Educational Psychology
Address: Faculty of Education, University of Colombo, Colombo 3, Sri Lanka.
E-mail: pgrsamudra@yahoo.com

## 7 References

Battle, J. (2002). *Culture-Free Self-Esteem Inventories Examiner's Manual.* Austin, TX: Pro-ED.

Bolhasan, R. B. A. (2009). A Study of Dyslexia Primary School Student in Malaysia. *European Journal, V*(1), 250–268.

Bruck, M. (1989). The adult outcomes of children with learning disabilities. *Annals of Dyslexia, 39*, 252–263.

Casey, R., Levy, S., Brown, K., & Brooks-Gunn, J. (1992). Impaired emotional health in children with mild reading disability. *Developmental and Behavioural Paediatrics, 13*, 256–260.

Eichhorn, R. (2016). Secondary Symptoms and Compensation Mechanism of Dyslexic Children. In E. Witruk, S. Novita., Y. Lee., & D. S. Utami (Eds.), *Studies in Educational and Rehabilitation Psychology: Dyslexia and Traumatic Experiences, Vol.7* (pp. 25–30). Frankfurt: Peter Lang.

Huntington, D. D., & Bender, W. N. (1993). Adolescents with learning disabilities at risk? Emotional well-being, depression, suicide. *Journal of Learning Disabilities, 26*(3), 159–166.

Katusic, S. K., Colligan, R. C., Barbaresi, W. J., Schaid, D. J., & Jacobsaon, S. J. (2001). Incidence of reading disability in a population based birth cohort 1976–1982 Rochester, Minn. *Mayo Clinic Proceedings, 76*, 1081–1092.

Paget, K. D., & Reynolds, C. R. (1984). Dimensions, levels and reliabilities on the revised children's manifest anxiety scale with learning disabled children. *Journal of Learning Disabilities, 17*, 137–141.

Senarath, S. (2016). Teachers' knowledge about the dyslexia. In E. Witruk, S. Novita., Y. Lee., & D. S. Utami (Eds.), *Studies in Educational and Rehabilitation Psychology: Dyslexia and Traumatic Experiences, Vol.7* (pp. 37–45). Frankfurt: Peter Lang.

Spence, S. H. (1998). A measure of anxiety symptoms among children. *Behavior Research and Therapy, 36*, 545–566.

Vigilante, F. W., & Dane, E. (1991). Teenage dyslexia: Stuerm und Drang. *Child and Adolescent Social Work, 8* (6), 515–523.

Willcutt, E. G., & Pennington, B. F. (2000). Psychiatric comorbidity in children and adolescents with reading disability. *Journal of Child Psychology and Psychiatry, 41*(8), 1039–1048.

Enoka Randeniya

# Comprehensive Reading Difficulties on Sinhala Language of Dyslexic Students in Sri Lanka

**Abstract:** According to the world declaration of "Education for All" that children, including children with dyslexia, have a right to education. In alignment with this, studies offering different perspectives on the education of dyslexic students have been carried out in many countries. However, only a very few research studies have been conducted in Sri Lanka. Also in Sri Lanka, teachers paid less attention to identifying students with dyslexia. Thus, this study attempts to investigate the comprehensive reading difficulties on the Sinhala language of dyslexic students in Sri Lanka. The study developed a qualitative research paradigm, adopting a multiple case study method and selecting a purposive sample of ten dyslexic students. Interviews, activity pack designed for the oral test, observations, medical reports of the dyslexic students and voice recordings of respondents were used for data collection. Data were analyzed and interpreted under five themes using within the case and cross-case analyzes, qualitatively as well as quantitatively. Findings of the study revealed that some common weaknesses exist in the comprehensive reading component of the language abilities as well as individual characteristics of each student in the sample. Under the five comprehensive reading difficulties investigated: (1) the ability to construct meaningful sentences declines when the number of words in a sentence is increasing, (2) grammatically correct sentences were able to construct only in present tense, (3) 60% of the sample successfully interpreted given symbols, (4) 70% of the sample was in satisfactory level of reading pictures replacing with appropriate words, and (5) answering questions given on a poem and a paragraph was in a poor level. These findings were informative to identify the comprehensive reading disabilities on the Sinhala language of dyslexic students and to implement relevant intervention methods to overcome comprehensive reading difficulties of dyslexic students.

**Keywords:** dyslexia, comprehensive reading difficulties, Sinhala language, purposive sample

## 1 Introduction

In align with the global challenges of the education, a higher level of children with a learning disability are increased. Dyslexia can be identified as a specific learning disability that manifests preliminarily as difficulty with learning to read. It is also neurobiological in origin. Dyslexia is characterized by problems with accurate and/or fluent word recognition and by poor spelling and decoding abilities (Lyon, 2003).

According to the International Statistical Classification of Diseases and Related Health Problems (ICD) 10th revision (World Health Organization [WHO], 2015), dyslexia follows as specific developmental disorders of scholastic skills, which is a specific and significant impairment in the development of reading skills that is not solely accounted by the mental age, visual acuity problems or inadequate schooling. Reading may be affected by reading comprehension skills, reading word recognition, oral reading skill, and performance of tasks requiring. This disorder is possible to exist in children with better, normal or average intelligence.

Modern research reveals that only intelligence quotient is not sufficient to assess dyslexics, but it is necessary to consider the cognitive processing skills to determine the dyslexics (Wang, Li, Georgiou, & Das, 2012). Hence, considering the diffusion of dyslexics, different prevalence rates can be seen all over the world such as 1% in Scandinavian countries and 3%-5% in Germany (Witruk, 2010). Studies related to different perspectives of dyslexia have been conducted in many countries based on the need of reducing the dropouts of dyslexics from the school setting. There is also a very few research studies related to dyslexia have been carried out in Sri Lankan context. Also Sri Lanka has accepted the world declaration on "Education for All" which states the necessity of providing basic education to all (The World Bank Group, 2000). Thus, to address the gap mentioned above in the field research of dyslexia in Sri Lanka, this study has been carried out under the main objective of identifying the comprehensive reading difficulties of dyslexics on the Sinhala language.

## 2 Theoretical Review

The review of literature of the study can be classified into two main categories; theoretical aspects and empirical research related to dyslexia. Several themes, namely definitions of dyslexia, cause for dyslexia, reading difficulties of dyslexics, and secondary characteristics of dyslexic students have been constructed based on the above-mentioned categories. The most accepted definition of dyslexia has been presented by the ICD-10 (2015), accordingly, dyslexia follows as specific developmental disorders of scholastic skills, which is a specific and significant impairment in the development of reading skills that are not solely accounted by the mental age, visual acuity problems or inadequate schooling. Reading comprehension skills, reading word recognition, oral reading skill, and performance of tasks requiring reading may be affected. Spelling difficulties are frequently associated with a specific reading disorder and often remain into adolescence even after some progress in reading has been made. Specific developmental disorders are commonly preceded by a history of disorders in speech and language development, associated emotional and behavioral disturbances are common during the school-age period.

Furthermore, the International Dyslexia Association (2003) and the British Dyslexia Association (2007) have also presented widely accepted definitions of dyslexia. Witruk (2010) defined dyslexia as a restricted developmental disorder in the acquisition of reading often connected with a disorder in an accusation of writing. According

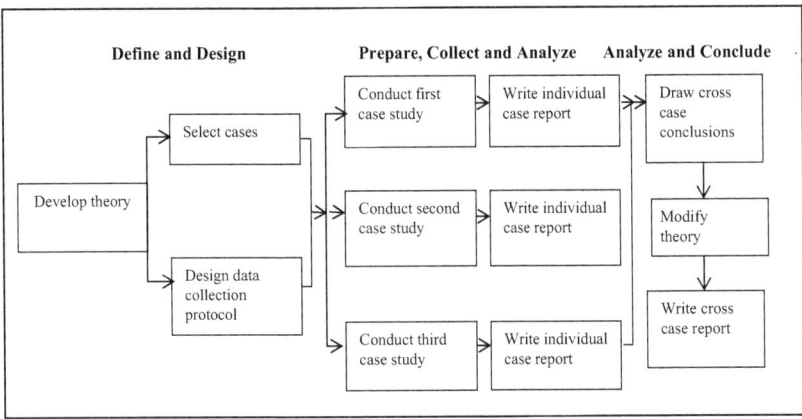

**Figure 1.** Case study method (Yin, 2009).

to the above definitions, dyslexia can be identified as a specific reading disability, including comprehensive reading skills. Causes of dyslexia can be identified based on the causal model (Morton, 2004) and multilevel model (Witruk, 1993) of dyslexia. Both models reveal that biological risk factors, i.e., genes preliminary cause of dyslexia. The left hemisphere of the brain of a dyslexic does not function properly as a result of distorted genes. This effects to make the phonological processing deficits in cognitive level and can be gradually seen from the behavioral characteristics, such as poor phonological awareness, inaccurate reading and spelling, and poor reading fluency. According to the multilevel model presented by Witruk (1993), reading and writing disabilities can emerge as primary symptoms of dyslexia, whereas partial performance deficits in perception, attention, memory, motor skills and integration works can be seen as secondary symptoms. Rispens (2004) highlighted the process of syntactic and phonological processing in developmental dyslexia. Moreover, this study revealed the different aspects related to reading acquisition: the phonological deficit theory, vocabulary development, and grammatical development.

# 3 Method

Under the qualitative research paradigm (see Figure 1), an exploratory multiple case study design was employed, based on the following diagram presented by Yin (2009).

## 3.1 Sample

Ten students who had been diagnosed with dyslexia by the Lady Ridgeway Hospital, Borella, Sri Lanka were purposively selected as the sample for the case study.

The sample consisted of eight boys and two girls those who studied in grade four (9 years) and five (10 years). Ethical clearance and parents' permission were obtained from the hospital and the parents before the selection of the sample.

### 3.2 Measurement Tools

The primary aim of this study was to investigate the comprehensive reading difficulties in the Sinhala language of dyslexic students in Sri Lanka. Different data collection and data analysing methods were used to achieve the objectives of the study. Interviews, observations, activity pack designed for the oral test, medical reports of the dyslexic students and voice recordings of respondents were used as data collection methods. The activity pack designed for oral test contained five items: 1) Construct meaningful sentences in order, 2) Construct grammatically correct sentences, 3) Reading by interpreting symbols, 4) Reading pictures are replacing with appropriate words, and 5) Answering questions given on a poem and a paragraph. Generated data were analyzed using within the case and cross-case analysis, qualitatively and quantitatively.

## 4 Results

This research intended to investigate the comprehensive reading difficulties on the Sinhala language of dyslexic students in Sri Lanka. Data collected under the five activities have been presented and analyzed as follows.

First activity attempted to measure the ability to construct meaningful sentences in order. There were seven sentences, and five of them consisted of less than six words, whereas the other two consisted of seven words. The remaining sentence consisted of twelve words. 80% of the sample constructed sentences in order when the sentences were consisted of less than six words and 30% of the sample constructed the sentences correctly when the sentence consisted of seven words. None of the students in the sample couldn't construct the final sentence in order which was consisted of twelve words. Furthermore, some of them have attempted more than once to construct the sentences in order, whereas some gave up after the first attempt.

The second activity was designed to construct grammatically correct sentences. There were five sentences to be built, according to the rules of Sinhala language. Then they had to select a verb according to the subject, considering the relevant tense. There were 70% of the students correctly constructed sentences given based on the first person present tense. More than 60% of the sample failed to construct sentences, given based on the second and third person as well as past and future tense. However, according to the observations, the respondents enjoyed participating activities and also expressed their personal experiences. None of the respondent students could correctly construct sentences according to the Sinhala grammar rule which requires to add an honorific ending (which is supposed to add a human quality to the noun) to an inanimate singular noun which will then be accompanied by a plural verb in a sentence.

The third activity was reading by interpreting symbols. There were four symbols which were graphical representatives of the words such as no smoking, poison, toilet and ladies only. There were 100% of the respondents correctly interpreted the symbol 'no smoking'. Furthermore, they identified the places where the 'no smoking' symbol is shown. More than 60% of the sample couldn't correctly interpret the symbols 'toilet' and 'ladies only'. Two students explained the graphical representations using English instead of Sinhala.

The fourth activity was to construct the story by reading pictures replacing the appropriate words. All students actively participated in this event, and two of them failed to replace the words instead of pictures. However, they have made some errors; omitted words or letters, substitution, mispronunciation, adding new words/letters, rapid naming problems and reading without stopping at the full stops in reading the story. The observations imply that the students enjoyed the activity a lot. One student has said that 'this story is very easy, isn't it?' All the students except one gave correct answers when some oral questions were asked based on the story.

Fifth activity was answering questions given in a poem and a paragraph. Four questions were given in the poem, and five questions were given under the paragraph. Two students gave correct answers to the questions based on the poem, four students gave incomplete answers, and the rest of the sample failed to give correct answers to all questions based on the poem. Even though they failed to answer correctly, it was observed that the students attempted their best to answer the questions. Anyone of the samples were unable to give correct answers to all the questions given based on the paragraph. Furthermore, four students couldn't give any correct answers to the questions based on the paragraph, and the rest of the sample provided incomplete answers. In addition to that, all the students made above mentioned common errors, in the fourth activity. Class teachers and parents also agreed with this situation of dyslexic students.

## 5 Conclusion

The first activity was to measure the ability to construct meaningful sentences. Considering the given answers by the students in the sample it could be observed that the ability to construct meaningful sentences declines when the number of words in a sentence is increasing. Mann, Shankwellier, and Smith (1984) also highlighted similar findings through their research. The second activity was to construct grammatically correct sentences. To give responses by the sample for this activity, a higher percentage of the sample failed to create correct sentences according to the subject of a second and third person as well as future and past tense. Casalis, Leuwer and Hilton (2012) presented the syntax while mentioning that reading is poor among dyslexic students. The third activity was reading by interpreting symbols. Even though all the students participated actively in the activity, all the students in the sample provided correct answers for at least two of the symbols. Based on their experimental research, Wolf and Obregon (1992) emphasised that the ability to read pictures of dyslexic children is higher when compared with other poor reading children. The next activity was, to construct the story by reading pictures replacing with appropriate words. A higher percentage of the sample have obtained a considerable level of achievement and actively participated in that event, expressing their ideas. Also, they were able to give answers orally. Fifth activity was answering questions provided in a poem and a paragraph. Even though a few students correctly answered the questions from the poem, all of them have failed to give correct answers to the questions provided in the paragraph. In addition to that, when reading the poem and the common paragraph errors were emerged. Casalis, Leuwers and Hilton (2012) conducted a research to identify the comprehensive reading difficulties on dyslexic students in France. It also scolded that comprehensive reading ability of the dyslexic students was poor compared to their chronological age.

As a summary, dyslexic students in Sri Lanka are suffering on comprehensive reading disability, and a few subcategories of dyslexics seems to be in different levels of reading. Therefore, government authorities related to the education need to get the necessary action to identify the unidentified dyslexic students and implement relevant intervention methods on dyslexics to overcome the Sinhala language reading disabilities. Also, parents and teachers should take their insight on how to interact with dyslexics without destroying their self-concept and teachers need to plan short term as well as long-term activity programs.

## 6 Affiliation

Dr. Enoka Randeniya
Institution/address: University of Colombo, Department of Educational Psychology, Faculty of Education, P. O. Box No. 1490, Cumaratunga Munidasa Mawatha, Colombo 3, Sri Lanka.
E-mail: erandeniya_m@yahoo.com

## 7 References

British Dyslexia Association. (2007). *Definition of Dyslexia*. Bracknell: BDA. Retrieved on March 16, 2018 from http://www.bdadyslexia.org.uk/about-dyslexia/further-information/dyslexia-research-information-html

Casalis, S., Leuwers, C., & Hilton, H. (2012). Syntactic Comprehension in Reading and Listening: A Study with French Children with Dyslexia. *Journal of Learning*, 46(3), 2010–2219.

International Dyslexia Association. (2010). *Knowledge and practice standards for teachers of reading*. Retrieved on March 5, 2018 from http://www.readingrockets.org/sites/default/files/IDA%20Knowledge%20and%20Practice%20Standards%20for%20Teaching%20of%20Reading.pdf

Lyon, G. G. (2003). A definition of dyslexia. *Annals of Dyslexia*, 53, 1–14.

Mann, V. A., Shankwellier, D. P., & Smith, S. T. (1984). The association between comprehension of spoken sentences and early reading ability: The role of phonitic representation. *Journal of Child Language*, 11, 627–643.

Morton, J. (2004). *Understanding developmental disorder: A causal model approach.* Oxford: Blackwell Publishing.

Rispens, J. E. (2004). *Syntactic and Phonological Processing in Developmental Dyslexia.* (Doctoral dissertation). Rijkuniversiteit Groningen, Netherland. Groningen: Print Partners Ipskamp Enschede. Retrieved on September 6, 2017 from https://www.researchgate.net/profile/Judith_Rispens/publication/30479925_Syntactic_and_phonological_processing_in_developmental_dyslexia/links/549027520cf225bf66a81de9/Syntactic-and-phonological-processing-in-developmental-dyslexia.pdf

Wang, X., George, K. G., Das, J. P., & Qing, L. (2012). Cognitive Processing Skills and Development Dyslexia in Chinese. *Journal of Learning Disabilities*, 45(6), 526–537.

Witruk, E. (1993). Memory Deficits of Dyslexic Children. In P. Tallal, M. A. Galaburda, R. Llinas, & C. von Euler (Eds.), *Temporal information processing in the nervous system. Special reference to dyslexia and dysphasia.* Annals of the New York Academy of Sciences, 682, (pp.430–435). New York: The New York Academy of Sciences.

Witruk, E. (2006, January). *Dyslexia-Assessment and Treatment.* Paper presented at the International Workshop Institute of Psychology II, University of Leipzig, Germany.

Witruk, E. (2010, January). *Dyslexia-Assessment and Treatment.* Paper presented at the International Workshop Institute of Psychology II, University of Leipzig, Germany.

Wolf, M., & Obregon, M. (1992). Early naming deficits, developmental dyslexia, and a specific deficit hypothesis. *Brain and Language*, 42(3), 219–247.

World Bank Group. (2000, April 26). *Education for all – from Jomtien to Dakar and Beyond.* Retrieved on August 4, 2017 from http://www.worldbank.org/

World Health Organization. (2015). *International Statistical Classification of Diseases and Related Health Problems 10th edition.* Retrieved on August 30, 2017 from http://apps.who.int/classifications/icd10/browse/2015/en

Yin, R. K. (2009). *Case Study research – Design and Methods* (4th Ed.). New Delhi: SAGE.

Francisca Serrano

# The Emotional Profile in Children with Dyslexia and Learning Disabilities

**Abstract:** Emotional features of dyslexia and other learning disabilities (LD) have been less studied than the cognitive or neural ones. However, there are severe emotional consequences coming from dyslexia and LD conditions, beyond those affecting to academic skills and behavior at the school, for example, frustration, anxiety to school activities or even depression, in more serious cases. These manifestations, often taken as secondary symptoms of dyslexia and LD, may be considered as primary problems if they develop to be more severe, affecting students' life not only at school but beyond in their personal or familiar circumstances. This paper reviews some research about emotional effects of dyslexia and LD, exploring the emotional profile in children with academic difficulties. It mainly focuses on the emotional variables self-concept, self-esteem and anxiety. This way it tries to contribute to a better understanding of the complexity behind dyslexia and LD manifestations.

**Keywords:** dyslexia, learning disabilities, self-concept, self-esteem, anxiety

## 1 Introduction

Cognitive, behavioral and neural features of dyslexia and other learning disabilities (LD) have been the main focus of psychological and educational research about these difficulties. Even existing definitions or the diagnostic criteria of these disorders in the Diagnostic and Statistical Manual of Mental Disorders fifth edition (DSM-5) (American Psychiatry Association [APA], 2013) principally describe cognitive and behavioral associated problems, do mention related neurobiological basis, but do focus less on consequences, especially of emotional nature.

Surely, serious consequences are coming from dyslexia and LD conditions, mainly affecting academic skills and behavior at the school. However, beyond that, very few are known and dyslexia and LD seem to stop being a problem once people are out of school or any academic/learning context (sometimes sadly due to school failure and dropout). Indeed, there is an agreement regarding the existence of other adverse effects out of those with academic nature, namely personal, emotional, motivational or familiar problems (Humphrey & Mullins, 2002). However, although acknowledged, they usually are taken as secondary symptoms, but not as a primary affectation (Novita, 2016). For that, it is expected that they will disappear after solving the academic problems, after overcoming them through psycho-educational intervention or once the students are out of the academic system.

But what happens when this is not the case, and these "secondary" effects continue affecting the individual's life? Sometimes they can bring severe impacts in the form of anxiety, frustration, depression, and behavioral problems with important consequences both in familiar and personal contexts and even in the clinical one when those effects concur with mental illness. Do they still have a secondary or a primary effect?

Unfortunately, research about emotional effects of LD is less extensive than that about cognitive or neural correlates. That can be due to the difficulty of studying them from a systematic research perspective. Available information comes from personal reports, parents' reports, qualitative questionnaires, and non-standardized measurement, all of them not without some bias for generalisation. Another obstacle for systematic research in the nature itself of these emotional variables. They usually do change over development or as a function of the testing moment, which make them non-stable constructs that could not be easily studied.

In any case, given the importance of the emotional manifestations or effects of LD, research about them is required. They cannot be ignored for any longer. To study them would contribute to a better understanding of these difficulties and in long-term, to the development of interventions for building a more stable emotional background for people with dyslexia and LD, encouraging high self-efficacy development beyond the school context.

This paper focuses on the emotional profile in children with dyslexia and LD aiming to review relevant information regarding this less studied topic. Moreover, it tries to go beyond studies and descriptions of the cognitive, neural and behavioral correlates of dyslexia and LD, thus increasing information available that it may be useful for developing more complete treatments in these difficulties. The combination of all information available will hopefully contribute to a better understanding of the complexity behind LD.

## 2 Emotional variables in dyslexia and LD

Dyslexia is defined by the DSM as a type of neuro-developmental disorder that causes problems for learning specific academic skills at the school context (i.e., reading, writing, or arithmetic) (DSM-5, APA, 2013); that is, it affects the basic skills for school learning. In that sense, it is considered a learning disability (LD), although these two terms (dyslexia and LD) cannot be taken as synonymous. Dyslexia's learning difficulties are 'unexpected' as other aspects of development seem not to be impaired. In that sense, it is considered as a specific learning disability (SLD). However, in the case of more general LD, there are normally other aspects of development affected, like oral language or cognitive skills like memory, attention or intelligence.

Besides this difference, both dyslexia and other LD share early signs of learning difficulties affecting reading and writing performance that may appear at the beginning of the school, generally in preschool (i.e., difficulty in phonological games, learning sequences, or names of letters). These problems continue through formal school, and they are typically detected in the 2nd or 3rd grade of primary school. Students with dyslexia and LD struggle to learn the correspondence between letters and sounds, show difficulties to decode single words either accurately or fluently, or both, read and write with effort and many mistakes, among other manifestations. As a consequence, they experience school failure; as the academic development advance without effective intervention, problems progressively increase, even leading to school dropout.

In this progress, the academic issues are usually accompanied by behavioral and emotional problems: frustration, the absence of discipline, emotional blockage, passive or aggressive attitudes, school refusal, feelings of inferiority, isolation, low self-concept and low self-esteem (Burden, 2008). These problems, regularly underestimated, can develop into more severe conditions concurring with anxiety, depression and learned helplessness regarding all school-related activities (Riddick, Sterling, Farmer, & Morgan, 1999). Overall, the situation becomes even more serious in the adolescence, in which self-esteem is the first element affected in case of school failure, which in turn affects the self-concept, which influences motivation (Carranza & Apaza, 2015).

However, there is still little research, and it is a topic that is necessary to be addressed (Humphrey, 2001; Riddick, 1996). There follows some evidence concerning emotional symptoms of dyslexia and LD, mainly focused on three of them: self-concept, self-esteem and anxiety.

## 3 Evidence about emotional symptoms of dyslexia and LD

The clinical experience and the qualitative research works indicate that the presence of dyslexia can determine a higher probability of psychological discomfort not only because the school activities can put the child at a disadvantage, but because they can bring a stressful position up compared to their classmates (Hellendoorn & Ruijssenaars, 2000). Some previous research has shown that children with dyslexia have low self-concept and self-efficacy (Bong & Skaalvik, 2003), low self-esteem (Polychroni, Koukoura & Anagnostou, 2006) and clinically significant levels of anxiety (Nelson & Harwood, 2011). But the characterization of these emotional variables remains unclear yet. Some relevant findings in this concern are reviewed below.

### 3.1 Self-concept

Self-concept is conceptualized as a multidimensional construct referred to the perception and the evaluation about oneself. Overall it includes a collection of beliefs about oneself, at different levels: cognitive, emotional, and behavioral. Moreover, it can be distinguished among academic, social and physical self-concept as a function of the necessary background considered.

Some studies have investigated the relationship between individual self-concept and academic achievement (Bong & Skaalvik, 2003), showing that low results at school will relate with little motivation for school's tasks which will lead to low self-concept.

Zeleke's meta-analysis (2004) regarding studies about self-concept and LD showed that most of the available research (89%) found lower academic self-concept in students with LD, compared to their peers without difficulties. Only 20% of the studies showed a lower social self-concept in people with LD, but 7% of the studies found the contrary result. And only 30% of the studies found a lower general self-concept in people with LD, compared to people without difficulties. Zeleke´s meta-analysis (2004) highlights the difficulties faced by research on this topic, and it proposes the convenience of different study levels of self-concept combined in one study.

For that reason, Ruz (2017) studied the different level of self-concept in the same study, which looked at academic, social, emotional, familiar aspects, together with the total measurement of self-concept.

Participants were 39 children, aged 8 to 12 years, studying primary school (3rd to 6th Grade). Twenty-three children had a diagnosis of dyslexia or LD (10 [43.5%] women; Mean age = 9.9 years, SD= 1.45). Professionals from the Pupil Guidance Center provided the diagnosis. They were compared to a control group of children without LD, attending the same classroom than children with dyslexia and LD and matched in age, sex and school level. The control group was compound of 16 children. Both groups did not differ in sex ($X^2(2, N = 39) < 0.001$; $p = 0.98$); Intelligence level - IQ ($t(37) = -1.26$; $p = 0.213$); or age ($t(39) = 0.74$; $p = 0.46$).

All students were tested with a self-concept standardised test AF5: Self-concept form 5 (AF-5; García & Musitu, 2014), evaluating different levels of self-concept: global, academic, social, familiar, and emotional.

Results showed that students with dyslexia and LD obtained lower results than their peers without academic difficulties not only in academic self-concept ($t(37) = -2.65$; $p = 0.012$), but also in the global measure of self-concept ($t(37) = -3.014$; $p = 0.003$) and in familiar self-concept ($t(37) = -2.85$; $p = 0.007$). There was also a tendency for lower results in emotional self-concept ($t(37) = -1.95$; $p = 0.058$) and no differences in social self-concept were found ($p > 0.05$). Figure 1 shows these results.

These findings support previous research about dyslexia, LD and Academic self-concept, but they also add evidence that may contribute to understanding the big picture. Students with difficulties get to have a lower perception about themselves in the academic level, after repeated failure at school. This perception affects not only to the academic level, but also get to affect to the familiar level, to the emotional one and overall, in a general way.

Therefore, students' problems in school do not only have consequences in the perception of themselves regarding the academic skills, but also they may affect their family. Some parents have reported a great variety of emotions related to the knowledge of their children as having LD: deception, frustration, fear, guilt, confusion. A high percentage (60%) even blame themselves for their children's difficulties, for not having detected them before or having looked for help earlier (for a review see Riddick, 2010). Consequences at the emotional level have also been

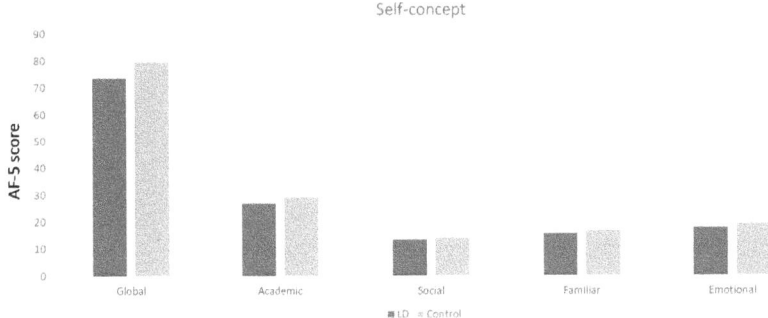

**Figure 1.** Mean score in different levels of self-concept (Global, Academic, Social, Familiar, and Emotional)

described; Hales (1994) showed how most of the children with LD at school experienced negative emotions like frustration, low motivation, and lack of confidence. However, social self-concept does not seem to be equally affected, but further investigation would be needed on the development of this self-concept dimension. Although young students inform that dyslexia or LD does not affect them to have friends out of school, how could the concept of themselves get affected through a life in which academic skills are so crucial for personal development? How could evolve this dimension through the adolescence or adult age?

Thus, there are still questions to be answered, for which research is needed.

## 3.2 Self-esteem

Self-esteem refers to the extent to which the perception about oneself match the image of how it should be or someone wants it to be. Thus, it is made of an individual's overall subjective emotional evaluation of his or her worth, and how does it make him or her feelings about it. Self-esteem would depend on the importance given to a specific domain (Burden, 2008). For example, if a student does not think that reading and writing are valuable skills, her/his academic self-esteem may not get affected by low performance in that skills at school. On the contrary, if she/he or someone important in their life (parents, teachers) thinks they are relevant skills, the self-esteem may get affected by low school scores in these skills.

Zuppardo, Serrano, & Pirrone (2017) carried out a preliminary assessment of the self-esteem in primary school children with dyslexia and LD, compared to that of children with no school problems. They followed the hierarchical self-esteem model, assuming that several dimensions associated with the multiple contexts where people act are equally important in building self-esteem, in general.

Participants were 25 students with dyslexia and dysorthographia (16 boys and nine girls). They had a previous diagnosis provided by professionals from the Pupil

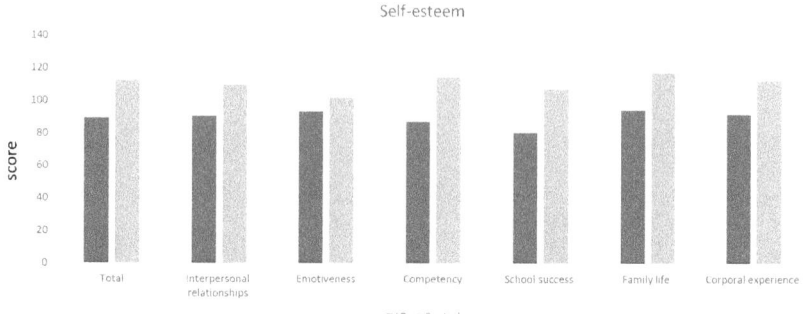

**Figure 2.** Mean score in different dimensions of self-esteem (Total, Interpersonal relationships, Emotiveness, Competency, Family life, and Corporal experience).

Guidance Center. They were compared with ten class-mates without learning problems (five boys and five girls). Age rate was among 8 and 18 years old, and they study Primary and Secondary school.

They were tested using the Bracken's Multidimensional Self-Esteem Assessment Test (Bracken, 1993), Italian version. The test considered six scales are matching the following self-esteem dimensions: Interpersonal relationships; Emotiveness; Competency/control over the environment; School success; Family life; Corporal experience; plus a total scale that provides information on the general self-esteem.

Results showed statistically significant differences between students with difficulties and their peers without them, in all self-esteem dimensions: Interpersonal relationships ($t = -6.04$; $p < 0.0001$); Emotiveness ($t = -2.83$ $p < 0.01$); Competency/control over the environment ($t = -6.90$; $p < 0.0001$); School success ($t = -7.20$; $p < 0.0001$); Family life ($t = -7.29$; $p < 0.0001$); Corporal experience ($t = -4.53$; $p < 0.0001$); and in the total scale ($t = -7.20$; $p < 0.0001$). Figure 2 shows these results, with lower scores in students with difficulties in all self-esteem dimensions, when compared to their colleagues without academic difficulties.

These findings support previous outcomes regarding self-concept, showing how poor performance in school has effects not only in the way individuals see themselves but also in the way they value this view. Moreover, it is evidenced how problems at school can influence emotional aspects like self-esteem, and not only in those dimensions closely related to schools, like competency and school success but beyond them in different extents like emotiveness and family life, as it was found regarding self-concept.

## 3.3 Anxiety

Mainly, anxiety is the most common emotional symptom in cases of dyslexia. Some studies (Nelson & Harwood, 2011) show the presence of symptoms

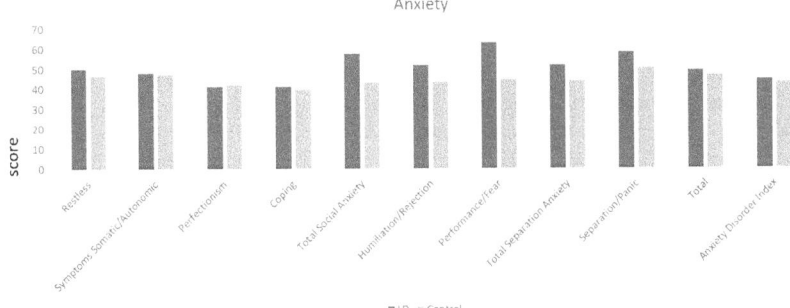

**Figure 3.** Mean score in different dimensions of the MASC - Physical symptoms (Restless and Somatic/Autonomic Symptoms); Avoidance (Perfectionism and Coping); Social Anxiety (Total score, Humiliation/Rejection, and Fear to public performance); Separation Anxiety (Total score and Separation/Panic); Total Anxiety score and Anxiety Disorder Index

attributable to school anxiety in around 70% of children with learning disorders. But what causes anxiety in people with dyslexia? What is behind of these anxiety problems?

For testing this, Zuppardo et al. (2017) also studied symptoms of anxiety in people with dyslexia and LD in school age, to determine the relevance of these symptoms and to what extent may they be related to school activities.

Participants (25 students with dyslexia and dysorthographia, compared to 10 class-mates without learning problems, as previously described) were tested using The Multi-dimensional Anxiety Scale for Children (MASC) (March, Parker, Sullivan, Stallings and Conner (1997). This test consists of 39 multiple response questions, and it measures if a child has a pathological anxiety condition (according to the DSM). It explores the following dimensions: Physical symptoms (Restless and Somatic/Autonomic Symptoms); Avoidance (Perfectionism and Coping); Social Anxiety (Total score, Humiliation/Rejection and Fear to public performance); Separation Anxiety (Total score and Separation/Panic); a total Anxiety score and the Anxiety Disorder Index (ADI).

Figure 3 shows the results in all dimensions both for children with difficulties and their peers without problems. Differences were statistically significant only in the total value of Social Anxiety ($t = 4.67$; $p = 0.001$) and in Fear to public performance ($t = 98.43$; $p = 0.001$). There were differences marginally significant in both dimensions of Separation Anxiety ($p = 0.06$) and Humiliation/Rejection ($p = 0.05$), another dimension of Social Anxiety.

Overall, anxiety symptoms in dyslexia appear to be related to Social Anxiety and Separation Anxiety dimensions. Moreover, these dimensions seem to be linked to typical school activities or situations. For example, the fear of public performance is often experienced when students have to present their work in front of the class orally. All students normally fear this activity, but it could be scarier for students with reading problems as he/she will need to read their work in front of everyone in the class. Humiliation or rejection could be experienced as a result of this type of activities. Actually, in some cases, there have been described cases of bullying in a population with dyslexia or LD, related to their problems at school (Livingston, Siegel, & Ribary, 2018).

# 4 Conclusion

Emotional aspects related to dyslexia and LD have been often underestimated, although they may play an important role in the evolution of the clinical picture of these academic difficulties. This paper highlights the need for studying emotional variables in a population with dyslexia and learning disabilities, aiming for improving their school performance and overall wellness.

Students with dyslexia and LD have shown to have a lower self-concept, self-esteem and higher levels of anxiety than their peers without academic difficulties, in school-related activities. These findings derive from systematic research using a standardised test, and not qualitative reports which were generally the source of previous data.

Overall, these emotional manifestations appear to be closely related to the problems at school. Academic self-concept seems more impaired than other self-concept dimensions. The same happens when examining self-esteem, being dimensions related to school success those in which students with dyslexia and LD show lower results than their colleagues. Equally, index of anxiety problems is found in school-related experiences, showing fear of making mistakes and being judged or not understood by others. Beyond them, emotional problems seem to spread in other extents like emotiveness and family life. As a consequence, these emotional problems could imply avoiding confrontation or potential success, not only during their time at school, but in different contexts (Hellendoorn & Ruijssenaars, 2000).

The emotional profile in students with dyslexia and LD should be considered at the same time of their learning difficulties because very often the stories of school failure do compromise not only the school but also personality development and social adjustment. Low self-concept, low self-esteem will lead to anxiety, sometimes leading to real depression and socialisation difficulties. For that, further research would be needed in other to study the interrelation among these emotional variables.

Positive emotions may be the foundation for adequate development at the social, academic or personal level and do play a crucial role in personality development (Idan & Margalit, 2014). To develop greater confidence in themselves and their capacities, knowing that each has its value should be part of treatment in dyslexia and LD.

## 5 Affiliation

Prof. Dr. Francisca Serrano
Institution: University of Granada
Address: Faculty of Psychology, Campus de Cartuja sn, Granada 18071, Spain
E-mail: fdserran@ugr.es

## 6 References

American Psychiatric Association (APA). (2013). *Diagnostic and statistical manual of mental disorders* (5th Ed.). Arlington, VA: APA.

Bong, M., & Skaalvik, E. M. (2003). Academic self-concept and self-efficacy: How different are they really? *Educational Psychologist Review, 15*(1), 1–40. https://doi.org/10.1023/A:1021302408382

Bracken, B. A. (1993). *Bracken's Multidimensional Self-Esteem Assessment Test.* Trent: Erikson.

Burden, R. (2008). Is dyslexia necessarily associated with negative feelings of self-worth? A review and implications for future research. *Dyslexia, 14* (3), 188–196. https://doi.org/10.1002/dys.371

Carranza, R. F., & Apaza, E. E. (2015). Academic self-concept and motivation in young talents of a private university in Tarapoto. *Journal of Educational Psychology-Propósitos y Representaciones, 3*(1), 249–263.

García, F., & Musitu, G. (2014). *AF-5. Autoconcepto Forma 5.* Madrid: TEA.

Hellendoorn, J., & Ruijssenaars, W. (2000). Personal experiences and adjustment of Dutch adults with dyslexia. *Remedial and Special Education, 21*(4), 227–239. doi:10.1177/074193250002100405

Humphrey, N. (2001). *Self-concept and self-esteem in developmental dyslexia: implications for teaching and learning* (Unpublished doctoral dissertation). Liverpool John Moores University, Liverpool.

Humphrey, N. & Mullins, M. P. (2002). Personal constructs and attribution for academic success and failure in dyslexia. *British Journal of Special Education, 29*(4), 196–203. https://doi.org/10.1111/1467-8527.00269

Idan, O., & Margalit, M. (2014). Socioemotional self-perceptions, family climate, and hopeful thinking among students with learning disabilities and typically achieving students from the same classes. *Journal of Learning Disabilities, 47*(2), 136–152. doi:10.1177/0022219412439608

Livingston, E. M., Siegel, L. S., & Ribary, U. (2018). Developmental dyslexia: emotional impact and consequences. *Australian Journal of Learning Difficulties,* 1–29. doi:10.1080/19404158.2018.1479975

March, J.S., Parker, J.D.A., Sullivan, K., Stallings, P. & Conners, C.K. (1997). The Multidimensional Anxiety Scale for Children (MASC): Factor structure, reliability, and validity. *Journal of the American Academy of Child and Adolescent Psychiatry, 36*, 554–565. doi:10.1097/00004583-199704000-00019

Nelson, J. M., & Harwood, H. (2011). Learning disabilities and anxiety: A meta-analysis. *Journal of Learning Disabilities, 44* (1), 3–17. doi:10.1177/0022219409359939

Novita, S. (2016). Secondary symptoms of dyslexia: A comparison of self-esteem and anxiety profiles of children with and without dyslexia. *European Journal of Special Needs Education, 31*(2), 279–288. doi:10.1080/08856257.2015.1125694

Polychroni, F., Koukoura, K., & Anagnostou, I. (2006). Academic self-concept, reading attitudes and approaches to learning of children with dyslexia: Do they differ from their peers? *European Journal of Special Needs Education, 21*(4), 415–430. doi:10.1080/08856250600956311

Riddick, B. (1996). *Living with dyslexia. The social and emotional consequences of special learning difficulties.* London: Routledge.

Riddick, B., Sterling, C., Farmer, M., & Morgan, S. (1999). Self-esteem and anxiety in the educational histories of adult dyslexic students. *Dyslexia, 5*(4), 227–248. https://doi.org/10.1002/(SICI)1099-0909(199912)5:4<227::AID-DYS146>3.0.CO;2-6

Ruz, A. (2017). *Autoconcepto y dyslexia* [Self-concept and dyslexia] (Unpublished bachelor thesis). University of Granada, Granada.

Zeleke, S. (2004). Self-concepts of students with learning disabilities and their normally achieving peers: A review. *European Journal of Special Needs Education, 19*(2), 145–170. doi:10.1080/08856250410001678469

Zuppardo, L., Serrano, F., & Pirrone, C. (2017). Delimitando el perfil emotivo-conductual en niños y adolescentes con dislexia [Outlining the emotional-behavioral profile in children and adolescent with dyslexia]. *Retos XXI, 1*(1), 88–104.

Isabel Leite & Tânia Fernandes

# A Dark Consequence of Developmental Dyslexia: Discrimination of Mirror Images is not Automatized

**Abstract:** Reading is a cultural activity too recent in the history of the humankind to be encrypted in the human genome but, paradoxically, some people fail to achieve fluent reading, despite adequate instruction and no sensorial or general cognitive deficits that could explain such specific difficulty. Intensive research has been devoted to the neurocognitive mechanisms of reading and the putative differences related to this specific developmental reading disorder or *dyslexia*. Much research has focused on the relation between literacy and oral language but reading is also an intensive visual activity that requires specific adaptations of the visual ventral system, including the suppression of *mirror invariance* (the perceptual bias by which one stimulus and its lateral reflection or mirror image, e.g., d and b, are processed as equivalent percept). Interestingly, *reversal* errors (e.g., confusing d with b) have long been documented in dyslexia. In the present paper, we review the available evidence regarding mirror-image processing in dyslexic children, taking into account the methodological aspects and shortcomings of prior studies. We also revisit our findings with typically-developing children (preliterate children and first grade beginning readers) and adults (illiterate, ex-illiterate, and schooled literate), and dyslexic children and their two control groups (of chronological age, and of reading level). Our research suggests that dyslexic readers fail to acquire the automatic changes promoted by literacy acquisition outside the written domain. More specifically, we argue that mirror-image discrimination, which is triggered by learning to read and occurs automatically in the course of visual object recognition in typically-developing readers, may never become automatised in dyslexic readers.

**Keywords:** literacy, developmental dyslexia, mirror invariance, mirror-image discrimination, visual processing

## 1 Introduction

In 1896, Morgan (1896) published one of the first scientific reports of a specific developmental reading disorder: The case of a 14-year-old boy that, despite adequate instruction and consistent educational experience, and no sensorial or general cognitive deficit, failed to acquire fluent automatic reading. Albeit with minor changes, this core definition of *developmental dyslexia* (henceforth, dyslexia) still applies (Peterson & Pennington, 2015). After more than 120 years of intensive research, important discoveries have been made on the neurocognitive mechanisms of reading and dyslexia (Martin, Kronbichler, & Richlan, 2016; Paulesu, Danelli, & Berlingeri, 2014; Vellutino, Fletcher, Snowling, & Scanlon, 2004), but a unified comprehensive framework is still lacking (Huettig, Lachmann, Reis, & Petersson, 2018; Lachmann & Geyer, 2003). This state of the art, as well as the (apparent) paradoxical observation of a specific disorder of a cultural acquired function, might be due to the fact that the changes promoted in evolutionary-older cognitive systems in the course of learning to read are not yet fully understood, being responsible for the heterogeneous profiles of dyslexia (Lobier & Valdois, 2015; Ramus, 2014; Vidyasgar & Pammer, 2010).

Literacy can be conceptualized as a bridge between two evolutionary-older cognitive systems that become highly interactive in the course of learning to read: visual object recognition and language (Dehaene & Cohen, 2011; Price & Devlin, 2011). A large amount of research has been devoted to the association between reading and phonological processing in both typical and dyslexic readers (Vellutino et al., 2004). Yet, reading is also an intensive visual activity with major consequences in occipital and occipitotemporal functioning due to highly demanding perceptual learning (Dehaene et al., 2010; Szwed, Dehaene, Kleinschmidt, Eger, Valabrègue, Amadon, & Cohen, 2011). It requires specific adaptations of the *ventral visual* system, which did not evolve for letter recognition and reading but rather for identification and categorisation of familiar objects (i.e., *vision-for-perception*) (Goodale & Milner, 1992).

## 2 Visual Object Recognition and Literacy

In recent years, an emergent bulk of research has examined the changes that learning to read promotes in the visual system, outside the written domain (Dehaene, Cohen, Morais, & Kolinsky, 2015), showing impacts in: (i) primary visual area (V1) functioning (Dehaene et al., 2010; Szwed, Qiao, Jobert, Dehaene, & Cohen, 2014); (ii) early perceptual processes such as feature integration (Szwed, Ventura, Querido, Cohen, & Dehaene, 2012); (iii) oculomotor control and selective visuospatial attention, as well as in the associated subcortical areas (Skeide et al., 2017); and (iv) the brain responses to other familiar visual categories in the ventral occipito-temporal cortex (vOT), such as to familiar objects and faces (Dehaene et al., 2010; Dundas, Plaut, & Behrmann, 2014).

When learning to read, letters become gears of words with features of a letter occurring adjacently to the features of neighbouring letters. To decode printing, high-resolution visual skills are necessary so that fast and accurate recognition of minute-difference symbols at specific positions within-words happens swiftly, while major low-level, non-diagnostic differences are disregarded (e.g., *e* and *c* are different letters, and *bone*, *done*, and *node* are different words, but *e* and *E*, and *node* and *NODE* are the same). Reading thus places high demands on visual processing (Grainger, 2018).

Most of the original properties of the vOT, part of the ventral visual pathway (Goodale & Milner, 1992), are ideally suited for letter and visual word recognition (e.g., preference for high-resolution central vision; sensitivity to line junctions; perceptual equivalence between different visual shapes, e.g., e = E, thanks to learning of arbitrary associations[22]). Nonetheless, some of the original properties of the vOT differ and even collide with those necessary for learning to read. Given this difference, examining the impact of literacy in these original properties is one of the most interesting ways to test the consequences of learning to read in visual object processing and to test the limits of brain plasticity promoted by this cultural acquisition.

## 3 Mirror Images and Literacy

One of the vOT properties that collides with learning scripts like the Latin alphabet or the Japanese kana is mirror-image generalization or *mirror invariance*: after familiarization with a symbol, e.g., d, its lateral reflection or mirror image, e.g., b, is processed as being the same percept (Bornstein, Gross, & Wolf, 1978; Dehaene, 2009). This bias for perceptual equivalence of mirror images seems to be rooted in evolution, given that natural objects are usually (quasi-) symmetric, and hence, processing the differences between two profile views (that is, mirror images) of the (same) object would slow down visual object recognition without any gain (Bornstein et al., 1978). Indeed, neuroimaging and behavioral studies have shown that mirror invariance is not only found in humans (Dehaene et al., 2010; Eger, Pinel, Dehaene, & Kleinschmidt, 2015; Kolinsky, Verhaeghe, Fernandes, Mengarda, Grimm-Cabral, & Morais, 2011; Pegado, Nakamura, Cohen, & Dehaene, 2011), especially children (Casey, 1984; Fernandes, Leite, Kolinsky, 2016; Gibson, Pick, Osser, & Gibson, 1962), but in several other species (Logothetis, Pauls, & Poggio, 1995; Rollenhagen & Olson, 2000; Scarf, Corballis, Güntürkün, & Colombo, 2017; Sutherland, 1960). However, when learning a script with such mirror-image symbols like b and d, mirror-image invariance needs to be suppressed so that these symbols can be discriminated and reading automatized.

Research in this domain, including ours, has shown that: (i) mirror-image discrimination is not a matter of development or maturation; (ii) mirror-image invariance is not an epiphenomenon of difficulties in orientation processing; (iii) discrimination of mirror images depends on learning a script with mirror-image symbols; (iv) it generalizes to other, -linguistic, visual categories; and (v) it becomes automatic in the course of visual object processing by readers of the Latin alphabet.

First, both preliterate children and *illiterate* adults (non-readers that did not learned to read because they never went to school just due to cultural, socioeconomic or political reasons) show difficulties in discrimination of mirror images (Kolinsky et al., 2011; Fernandes et al., 2016; Fernandes & Kolinsky, 2013), which are no longer found in 1st-grade beginning readers or ex-*illiterate* adults (who learned to read in alphabetization courses during adulthood). Second, both preliterate children and illiterate adults are quite able to discriminate other orientation contrasts, as long as these correspond to rotations in the image plane (e.g., 90°, *N* and *Z*; 180°, *d* and *p* (Fernandes et al., 2018)); for these *plane* rotations, non-readers are as able to attend to orientation as to visual shape (Fernandes et al., 2016; Fernandes & Kolinsky, 2013; Kolinsky & Fernandes, 2014). These empirical findings agree with the observation that the vOT is sensitive to plane rotations but not to mirror images (Logothetis et al., 1995; Rollenhagen & Olson, 2000), and hence, mirror-image invariance is specific and not a mere epiphenomenon of a general difficulty in orientation processing. Third, learning to read is not enough for overcoming mirror invariance: Mirror-image discrimination is triggered by learning a script with mirror-image symbols. Readers of Tamil, a script without mirror-image symbols, show difficulties in mirror-image discrimination (Danziger & Pederson, 1998; Pederson, 2003) just like preliterate children or illiterate adults do (Kolinsky et al., 2011; Fernandes et al., 2016). Forth, mirror-image discrimination (promoted by learning a script with mirror-image symbols) generalizes to other visual categories, either of novel objects (e.g., blob-like shapes (Kolinsky et al., 2011)) or of familiar ones, like pictures of cloth, tools, or faces (Pegado et al., 2014). Finally, learning to read comes at a cost in visual object recognition. In fact, during visual object processing by readers, mirror-image discrimination occurs automatically even when it is irrelevant to the task (Kolinsky & Fernandes, 2014; Pegado et al., 2014): When participants are asked to decide whether two stimuli have the same or a different shape, only readers show worse performance for mirror-image (e.g., d and b) than for identical (d and d) pairs. Remarkably, in this *shape-based* task, preliterate children are significantly faster than 1st-grade children exclusively for mirror-image pairs (Fernandes et al., 2016). After just eight-months of literacy instruction, beginning readers already show one of the visual adaptations resulting from literacy acquisition. In fact, at the individual level, insipient mirror discrimination can be seen even before formal literacy instruction (Kolinsky & Fernandes, 2014). Sensitivity to mirror-image differences is strongly associated with letter knowledge in preliterate children (Fernandes et al., 2016): The better their letter knowledge, the stronger the interference on shape-based judgments for mirror-image relative to identical pairs and the least their difficulty in explicit mirror-image discrimination.

It thus seems surprising that reversals errors (e.g., confusing b with d) have long been documented in developmental dyslexia (Graveson & Standing, 1986; Kaltner & Jansen, 2014; Lyle & Goyen, 1968; Orton, 1928; Terepocki, Kruk, & Willows, 2002; Wolff & Melngailis, 1996) (for a recent review, see Fernandes & Leite, 2017), given that in typically-developing preliterate children, insipient mirror-image discrimination can already be observed allied with high letter knowledge (Fernandes et al., 2016). In 2017, we thus investigated the cause of reversals in developmental dyslexia (Fernandes & Leite, 2017).

## 4 Reversal Errors and Developmental Dyslexia

Reversal errors are frequent in the first years of reading in typically-developing children (Casey, 1986; Cornell, 1985; Frith, 1971; Gibson, Pick, Osser, & Gibson, 1962) and seem to be predominant and last for longer in readers with dyslexia (Terepocki et al., 2002). This difficulty in discriminating mirror-image letters could actually have the same origin as the paradoxical result reported by Lachman and van Leeuwen (2007): in a shape-based task (in which orientation-contrast pair of the same shape should be judged as same, disregarding the orientation differences) dyslexic children performed better and faster than chronologically-age control readers (i.e., CAC). At the group level, this pattern of results was quite similar to the one we have later found in typically-developing preliterate children (Fernandes et al., 2016) (for similar results with illiterate adults, see Kolinsky & Fernandes, 2014; Pegado et al., 2014). Whereas at first sight, the pattern of results of Lachman and van Leeuwen (2007) seemed due to low reading experience by dyslexic children, rather than causally associated with the reading disorder, we showed that the results were not as simple as that (Fernandes & Leite, 2017).

To provide a complete scenario, our study was grounded on four methodological pillars. First, to test whether the putative difficulty in mirror-image discrimination of dyslexic children was causally related with the reading disorder or (mere) consequence of reading level, besides dyslexic children, not only a CAC group but also a younger typically-developing group with the same reading level as dyslexics, that is, reading-level controls (RLC), was examined (Goswami, 2003). Second, to test whether this difficulty was mere expression of a general difficulty in orientation processing (Graveson & Standing, 1986; Kaltner & Jansen, 2014; Terepocki et al., 2002), besides mirror images, another orientation-contrast was examined, one in which typically-developing participants do not show difficulties of discrimination, regardless of their reading skills (Fernandes et al., 2016; Fernandes & Kolinsky, 2013; Kolinsky et al., 2011). Two types of orientation-contrasts were thus considered with the same 180° angular difference between members of a pair: mirror images (e.g., d and b) and plane rotations (e.g., d and p). Third, to explore whether the putative difficulty of dyslexics was specific to the written code, participants were presented with single letters and geometric-like shapes (matched in visual complexity). Finally, to examine whether mirror-image discrimination becomes as automatic in dyslexic as in typical readers in the course of learning to read, we analyzed their performance with mirror-image pairs in two tasks: when orientation was the task-criterion, in the orientation-based task; when orientation was irrelevant to the task, in the shape-based task. Dyslexic children were as good as RLC in explicitly discriminating mirror-image pairs, and both groups were worse than CAC. However, dyslexic children did not show the automatization of mirror-image discrimination that both CAC and the younger RLC showed. This pattern of the result was not specific to letters; it was found overall, for both letters and geometric-like shapes. To put it simply, in the vein of Lachmann and van Leeweun (2007), dyslexic children did not show any interference on shape-based judgments of mirror-image relative to identical pairs, in contrast to typical readers. These results thus show that dyslexic readers did not automatically process the mirror-image differences in the course of object recognition, which might seem to resemble the results found in typically-developing non-readers. However, this is not correct: Note that, although at the group level, for both illiterate adults and preliterate children, mirror-discrimination was hard and did not occur automatically, their letter knowledge (in the absence of decoding abilities) was associated with mirror-discrimination abilities.

In contrast, for dyslexics, despite years of reading instruction, mirror-discrimination was not yet automatic, probably because the functional changes promoted by literacy (which in typical readers are automatized), in dyslexic readers are not consolidated. Therefore, our position is that the deficit observed in the automatic mirror-image processing in dyslexia could reflect difficulties in long-term neurocognitive plasticity regarding the emergence of the reading circuitry and, consequently, on the effects that reading would have in other cognitive systems outside the written domain. From this proposal, we would also expect that any other adaptation, promoted by learning to read, which departs from the original properties of the evolutionary-older systems (in language and/or in object recognition) would show the same deviant path in developmental dyslexia.

We found consistent results along this prediction for another visual adaptation required when learning to read (Fernandes, Vale, Martins, Morais, & Kolinsky, 2014). For efficient letter and visual word recognition, letters must become significantly immune to interference from adjacent stimuli. In contrast to other objects, letters usually occur within strings in strong conditions of crowding (Grainger, Tydgat, & Isselé, 2010; Tydgat & Grainger, 2009) (for a review, see Grainger, 2017). In contrast to other stimuli (e.g., symbols as %, $), letters show minimal inter-letter interference. Reduced crowding holds for both single letters and letters within-strings recognised by either child or adult readers (Lachmann & van Leeuwen, 2007; Grainger et al., 2010; Ziegler, Pech-Georgel, Dufau, & Grainger, 2010). Whereas the recognition of a letter (e.g., *A*) is immune to the surrounding information, even if inserted in an enclosing shape, regardless of visual similarity (similar performance when *A* is surrounded by a square or a triangle), non-letters show congruence effects (i.e., better performance when surrounded by similar than dissimilar shapes). This differential congruence effect is specific to non-letters and not found for letters, for 8- and 10- year-olds and adult readers, and even for illiterate adults. Indeed, not only at the group level illiterates did not show a congruence effect for letters (only for non-letters), but at the individual level the larger their letter knowledge, the smaller the congruence effect for letters. Interestingly, and again despite years of literacy instruction, dyslexic children fail to show immunity to the surrounding information when recognising letters: They presented congruence effects for both letters and non-letters. Thus, it could be that these two difficulties, that is mirror-image processing and in inter-letter interference have the same foci.

## 5 Conclusion

Literacy acts as a bridge between two evolutionary-older systems. Visual object recognition and oral language are close to the novel function and sufficiently plastic to be partially re-oriented to allow the emergence of a highly specialised reading circuitry (Dehaene, 2009). Given the long history of reversal errors in dyslexia, the study of this (and other) visual adaptation(s), consequent of learning to read, is an interesting way to explore whether less flexibility or less consolidation of these changes could be causally related with the specific reading disorder.

Our results, together with previous findings, show that mirror discrimination is not a precondition for learning to read. The comparison between mirror-discrimination abilities of non-readers (illiterate adults and preliterate children) and readers (ex-illiterate and literate adults and child readers) has clearly shown that mirror discrimination depends on learning to read in a script with mirror-image symbols and that in typical readers little reading experience is sufficient to suppress mirror invariance. Indeed, typical readers from the 1st-, 3rd, and 5th-grader automatically discriminate left-right differences, even when deleterious for the current task. The difference in mirror-image discrimination between these typical readers and dyslexic children (Fernandes et al., 2016; Fernandes & Leite, 2017) can thus hardly be due to reduced/suboptimal reading experience (Huettig et al., 2018). We believe that it possibly reflects limits of brain plasticity (either in emergence or consolidation of the long-term changes promoted by literacy). In the quest for a possible comprehensive explanation of developmental dyslexia, one inevitable question is whether difficulties in neurocognitive plasticity (like those associated with sleep patterns, see Bruni et al., 2009) could ground the (apparent) heterogeneity of profiles previously reported in the specific reading disorder.

# 6 Affiliations

Prof. Dr. Isabel Leite
Institution: University of Évora
Address: Departmento de Psicologia, Colégio Pedro da Fonseca, Universidade de Évora, Apartado 94, 7002-554 Évora, Portugal.
E-mail: imss@uevora.pt

Prof. Dr. Tânia Fernandes
Institution: Faculdade de Psicologia, Universidade de Lisboa
Address: Alameda da Universidade, 1649-013 Lisboa, Portugal
E-mail: tpfernandes@psicologia.ulisboa.pt

# 7 Acknowledgement

This work has been supported by the Research Center in Psychological Science of Universidade de Lisboa (CICPSI) and by the scientific project VOrtEx, ref C490630733-00081487 (nº 28184) funded by Fundação para a Ciência e Tecnologia, FCT (02/SAICT/2017), Ministry of Science, Technology and Higher Education, Portugal.

# 8 References

Bornstein, M. C., Gross, C. G., & Wolf, J. Z. (1978). Perceptual similarity of mirror images in infancy. *Cognition*, 6(2), 89–116. doi: 10.1016/0010-0277(78)90017-3.

Bruni, O., Ferri, R., Novelli, L., Terribili, M., Troianiello, M., Finotti, E., ... Curatolo, P. (2009). Sleep spindle activity is correlated with reading abilities in developmental dyslexia. *Sleep*, 32 (10), 1333–1340. doi: 10.1093/sleep/32.10.1333

Casey, M. B. (1984). Individual differences in use of left–right visual cues: A reexamination of mirror-image confusions in preschoolers. *Developmental Psychology*, 20, 551–559. doi:10.1037/0012-1649.20.4.551

Casey, M. B. (1986). Individual differences in selective attention among prereaders: A key to mirror-image confusions. *Developmental Psychology*, 22, 58–66.

Cornell, J. M. (1985). Spontaneous mirror-writing in children. *Canadian Journal of Psychology-Revue Canadienne De Psychologie*, 39, 174–179.

Danziger, E., & Pederson, E. (1998). Through the looking- glass: Literacy, writing systems and mirror-image discrimination. *Written Language and Literacy*, 1, 153–164.

Dehaene, S. (2009). *Reading in the brain: The new science of how we read*. New York: Penguin.

Dehaene, S., & Cohen, L. (2011). The unique role of the visual word form area in reading. *Trends in Cognitive Sciences*, 15(6), 254–262. doi:10.1016/j.tics.2011.04.003

Dehaene, S., Cohen, L., Morais, J., & Kolinsky, R. (2015). Illiterate to literate: behavioural and cerebral changes induced by reading acquisition. *Nature Reviews. Neuroscience*, 16(4), 234–244. doi: 10.1038/nrn3924

Dehaene, S., Pegado, F., Braga, L. W., Ventura, P., Nunes Filho, G., Jobert, A., ... Cohen L. (2010). How Learning to Read Changes the Cortical Networks for Vision and Language. *Science*, 330, 1359. doi: 10.1126/science.1194140

Dundas, E. M., Plaut, D. C., & Behrmann, M. (2014). Variable Left-hemisphere Language and Orthographic Lateralization Reduces Right-hemisphere Face Lateralization. *Journal of Cognitive Neuroscience*, 27(5), 913–925. doi:10.1162/jocn_a_00757

Eger E., Pinel P., Dehaene S., & Kleinschmidt A. (2015). Spatially invariant coding of numerical information in functionally defined subregions of human parietal cortex. *Cerebral Cortex*, 25(5), 1319–1329. doi: 10.1093/cercor/bht323

Fernandes, T., & Kolinsky, R. (2013). From hand to eye: The role of literacy, familiarity, graspability, and vision-for-action on enantiomorphy. *Acta Psychologica*, 142, 51–61. doi:10.1016/j.actpsy.2012.11.008

Fernandes, T., & Leite, I. (2017). Mirrors are hard to break: A critical review and behavioral evidence on mirror-image processing in developmental dyslexia. *Journal of Experimental Child Psychology*, 159, 66–82. doi: 10.1016/j.jecp.2017.02.003

Fernandes, T., Coelho, B., Lima, F., & Castro, S. L. (2018). The handle of literacy: evidence from preliterate children and illiterate adults on orientation discrimination of graspable and non-graspable objects. *Language, Cognition and Neuroscience*, 33(3), 278–292. doi:10.1080/23273798.2017.1283424

Fernandes, T., Leite, I., & Kolinsky, R. (2016). Into the looking glass: Literacy acquisition and mirror invariance in preschool and first-grade children. *Child Development*, 87(6), 2008–2025. doi: 10.1111/cdev.12550

Fernandes, T., Vale, A. P., Martins, B., Morais, J., & Kolinsky, R. (2014). The deficit of letter processing in developmental dyslexia: combining evidence from dyslexics, typical readers and illiterate adults. *Developmental Science*, 17, 125–141. doi:10.1111/desc.12102

Frith, U. (1971). Why do children reverse letters? *British Journal of Psychology*, 62, 459–468. doi: 10.1111/j.2044-8295.1971.tb02059.x

Gibson, E. J., Pick, A. D., Osser, H., & Gibson, J. J. (1962). A developmental study of discrimination of letter-like forms. *Journal of Comparative and Physiological Psychology*, 55, 897–906. doi:10.1037/h0043190

Goodale, M. A., & Milner, A. D. (1992). Separate visual pathways for perception and action. *Trends in Neurosciences*, 15, 20–25. doi: 10.1016/0166-2236(92)90344-8

Goswami, U. (2003). Why theories about developmental dyslexia require developmental designs. *Trends in Cognitive Sciences*, 7, 534–540. doi: 10.1016/j.tics.2003.10.003

Grainger, J. (2017). Orthographic processing: A "mid-level" vision of reading. Quarterly *Journal of Experimental Psychology, 71*(2), 335–359. doi:10.1080/17470218.2017.1314515

Grainger, J. (2018). Orthographic processing: A "mid-level" vision of reading: The 44th Sir Frederic Bartlett Lecture. *Quarterly Journal of Experimental Psychology*, 71(2), 335–359. doi: 10.1080/17470218.2017.1314515

Grainger, J., Tydgat, I., & Isaclé, J. (2010). Crowding affects letters and symbols differently. *Journal of Experimental Psychology: Human Perception and Performance*, 36 (3), 673–688. doi: 10.1037/a0016888

Graveson, L., & Standing, L. (1986). Recognition of form and of orientation by poor and normal readers. *Perceptual and Motor Skills*, 63, 735–741. doi: 10.2466/pms.1986.63.2.735

Hoffman, K. L. & Logothetis, N. K. (2009). Cortical mechanisms of sensory learning and object recognition. *Philosophical Transactions of the Royal Society*, B (364), 321–329. doi: 10.1098/rstb.2008.0271

Huettig, F., Lachmann, T., Reis, A., & Petersson, K. M. (2018). Distinguishing cause from effect - Many deficits associated with developmental dyslexia may be a consequence of reduced and suboptimal reading experience. *Language, Cognition and Neuroscience*, 33(3), 333–350. doi:10.1080/23273798.2017.1348528

Kaltner, S., & Jansen, P. (2014). Mental rotation and motor performance in children with developmental dyslexia. *Research in Developmental Disabilities*, 35, 741–754. doi: 10.1016/j.ridd.2013.10.003

Kolinsky, R., & Fernandes, T. (2014). A cultural side effect: Learning to read interferes with identity processing of familiar objects. Special Issue: The impact of learning to read on visual processing. *Frontiers in Psychology*, 5, 1224. doi:10.3389/fp- syg.2014.01224

Kolinsky, R., Verhaeghe, A., Fernandes, T., Mengarda, E. J., Grimm-Cabral, L., & Morais, J. (2011). Enantiomorphy through the looking glass: Literacy effects on mirror-image discrimination. *Journal of Experimental Psychology: General*, 140, 210–238. doi:10.1037/A0022168

Lachmann, T., & Geyer, T. (2003). Letter reversals in developmental dyslexia: Is the case really closed? A critical review and conclusions. *Psychology Science*, 45, 53–75.

Lachmann, T., & Van Leeuwen, C. (2007). Paradoxical enhance- ment of letter recognition in developmental dyslexia. *Developmental Neuropsychology*, 31(1), 61–77. doi:10.1207/ s15326942dn3101_4.

Lobier, M., & Valdois, S. (2015). Visual attention deficits in developmental dyslexia cannot be ascribed solely to poor reading experience. *Nature Review Neuroscience*, 16(4), 225–225. doi:10.1038/nrn3836-c1

Logothetis, N. K., Pauls, J., & Poggio, T. (1995). Shape representation in the inferior temporal cortex of monkeys. *Current Biology*, 5, 552–563. doi: 10.1016/S0960-9822(95)00108-4

Lyle, J. G., & Goyen, J. (1968). Visual recognition, development lag, and strephosymbolia in reading retardation. *Journal of Abnormal Psychology*, 73(1), 25–29. doi: 10.1037/h0025458

Martin, A., Kronbichler, M., & Richlan, F. (2016). Dyslexic Brain Activation Abnormalities in Deep and Shallow Orthographies: A Meta-Analysis of 28 Functional Neuroimaging Studies. *Human Brain Mapping*, 37(7), 2676–2699. doi:10.1002/hbm.23202

Orton, S. T. (1928). Specific reading disability—Strephosymbolia. *Journal of the American Medical Association*, 90, 1095–1099. .doi: 10.1001/jama.1928.0269041000700

Paulesu, E., Danelli, L., & Berlingeri, M. (2014). Reading the dyslexic brain: multiple dysfunctional routes revealed by a new meta-analysis of PET and fMRI activation studies. *Frontiers in Human Neuroscience*, 8(830). doi:10.3389/fnhum.2014.00830

Pederson, E. (2003). Mirror-image discrimination among nonliterate, monoliterate, and biliterate Tamil subjects. *Written Language and Literacy*, 6, 71–91. doi:10.1075/ wll.6.1.04ped

Pegado, F., Nakamura, K., Braga, L. W., Ventura, P., Filho, G. N., Pallier, C. ... Dehaene, S. (2014). Literacy Breaks Mirror Invariance for Visual Stimuli: A Behavioral Study with Adult Illiterates. *Journal of Experimental Psychology: General, 143*(2), 887–894. doi: 10.1037/a0033198

Pegado, F., Nakamura, K., Cohen, L., & Dehaene, S. (2011). Breaking the symmetry: Mirror discrimination for single letters but not for pictures in the visual word form area. *Neuro Image*, 55, 742–749. doi:10.1016/j.neuroimage.2010.11.043

Peterson, R. L., & Pennington, B. F. (2015). Developmental dyslexia. *Annual Review of Clinical Psychology*, 11, 283–307. doi: 10.1146/annurev-clinpsy-032814-112842

Price, C. J., & Devlin, J. T. (2011). The interactive account of ventral occipitotemporal contributions to reading. *Trends in Cognitive Sciences, 15*(6), 246–253. doi:10.1016/j.tics.2011.04.001

Pringle Morgan, W. (1896). A Case of Congenital Word Blindness. *British Medical Journal, 2*(1871), 1378–1378.

Ramus, F. (2014). Neuroimaging sheds new light on the phonological deficit in dyslexia. *Trends in Cognitive Sciences, 18*(6), 274–275. doi:10.1016/j.tics.2014.01.009

Rollenhagen, J. E., & Olson, C. R. (2000). Mirror-image confusion in single neurons of the macaque inferotemporal cortex. *Science*, 287, 1506–1508. doi: 10.1126/science.287.5457.1506

Scarf, D., Corballis, M. C., Güntürkün, O., & Colombo, M. (2017). Do 'literate' pigeons show mirror-word generalization? *Animal Cognition, 20*(5), 999–1002. doi: 10.1007/s10071-017-1116-4

Skeide, M. A., Kumar, U., Mishra, R. K., Tripathi, V. N., Guleria, A., Singh, J. P., .. . Huettig, F. (2017). Learning to read alters cortico-subcortical cross-talk in the visual system of illiterates. *Science Advances, 3*(5). doi:10.1126/sciadv.1602612

Sutherland, N. S. (1960). Visual discrimination of orientation by octopus: mirror images. *British Journal of Psychology*, 51, 9–18. doi: 10.1111/j.2044-8295.1960.tb00719.x

Szwed, M., Dehaene, S., Kleinschmidt, A., Eger, E., Valabrègue, R., Amadon, A., & Cohen, L. (2011). Specialization for written words over objects in the visual cortex. *NeuroImage, 56*(1), 330–344. doi: 10.1016/j.neuroimage.2011.01.073.

Szwed, M., Qiao, E., Jobert, A., Dehaene, S., & Cohen, L. (2014). Effects of Literacy in Early Visual and Occipitotemporal Areas of Chinese and French Readers. *Journal of Cognitive Neuroscience, 26*(3), 459–475.doi: 10.1162/jocn_a_00499

Szwed, M., Ventura, P., Querido, L., Cohen, L., & Dehaene, S. (2012). Reading acquisition enhances an early visual process of contour integration. *Developmental Science*, 15, 139–149. doi:10.1111/j.1467-7687.2011.01102.x

Terepocki, M., Kruk, R. S., & Willows, D. M. (2002). The incidence and nature of letter orientation errors in reading disability. *Journal of Learning Disabilities*, 35, 214–233. doi: 10.1177/002221940203500304

Tydgat, I., & Grainger, J. (2009). Serial position effects in the identification of letters, digits and symbols. *Journal of Experimental Psychology: Human Perception and Performance*, 35(2), 480–498. doi:10.1037/a0013027

Vellutino, F. R., Fletcher, J. M., Snowling, M. J., & Scanlon, D. M. (2004). Specific reading disability (dyslexia): What have we learned in the past four decades? *Journal of Child Psychology and Psychiatry*, 45(1), 2–40. doi:10.1046/j.0021-9630.2003.00305.x

Vidyasagar, T. R., & Pammer, K. (2010). Dyslexia: a deficit in visuo-spatial attention, not in phonological processing. *Trends in Cognitive Sciences*, 14(2), 57–63. doi:10.1016/j.tics.2009.12.003

Wolff, P. H., & Melngailis, I. (1996). Reversing letters and reading transformed text in dyslexia: A reassessment. *Reading and Writing*, 8, 341–355.

Ziegler, J. C., Pech-Georgel, C., Dufau, S., & Grainger, J. (2010). Rapid processing of letters, digits and symbols: what purely visual-attentional deficit in developmental dyslexia? *Developmental Science*, 13(4), 8–14. doi: 10.1111/j.1467-7687.2010.00983.x

Adil Ishag

# The Impact of Diglossia on Arabic Reading Comprehension

**Abstract:** Diglossia emerges in a situation where two distinct varieties of a language are used alongside within a particular community. In this case, one is considered as a high or standard variety and the second one as a low or colloquial variety. Arabic is an extreme example of a highly diglossic language due to complexity in orthography and cursive consonant script. Lack of representation of short vowels in the alphabet is also Arabic idiosyncratic, which further negatively affects basic literacy skills attainment and contributes to the difficulty of reading comprehension tasks in Arabic. This article tries to conceptualize the notion of diglossia and its functions and characteristics. It further investigates the diglossic nature of Arabic and its impact on literacy attainment and reading comprehension process about the writing system, by scrutinising some empirical studies and relevant literature in the field.

**Keywords:** diglossia, standard Arabic, literacy acquisition, reading comprehension

## 1 Introduction

Diglossia is a sociolinguistic term that was reconceptualized by Ferguson in 1959, referring to a situation in which two varieties of a language exist side by side throughout the community, with each having a definite role to play. Ferguson identified four languages as being diglossic namely; Arabic, Greek, Haitian Creole, and Swiss German. The two varieties of any diglossic language co-exist alongside each other within a single community, one functioning as a standard and high variety (H) and the second one as a low variety (L). Therefore, diglossia essentially differs from bilingualism which refers to co-existence of entirely two different languages. Fishman (1970) further expanded Ferguson's original notion of diglossia and distinguished between bilingualism and diglossia by stating that bilingualism is an essential characterization of linguistical versatility, whereas diglossia is a characterization of the societal allocation of functions to different varieties of languages. Thus, it suggests that diglossia emerges within a language speaking community and as such, it is collectivistic, while bilingualism mostly refers to an individual's ability to communicate in two languages.

Diglossia is recognised by some characteristics and features as follows:

a) Stability: Diglossia is a relatively stable sociolinguistic situation that persists for a long period, which is also the case of Arabic diglossia that dates back to a few centuries, in which various Arabic dialects emerged alongside classical Arabic.

b) Complexity: The standard and high variety are thought to be more complex regarding the grammatical, stylistic and syntactic system than the low variety. For instance, vernacular Arabic is considered to be less linguistically sophisticated than standard or classical Arabic.
c) Functions and prestige: One of the most identifying features of diglossia is using the two varieties to serve different functions, in which the high variety is used in formal settings such as broadcasting, schooling, mosques and official ceremonies, while the low variety is used in everyday communication. Regarding prestige, the standard and high variety is usually deemed to be more prestigious and has a higher status than the common and low variety; this might be because classical Arabic is the language of the Quran. According to Palmer (2007), spoken vernacular Arabic is often stigmatised and considered less prestigious and as such there are few investigations on spoken colloquial Arabic, although it is the language of daily communication and widely used than standard Arabic.
d) Standardisation: The high variety is standardised and has a written form that is unified across the Arab world in formal discourse, whereas the low variety lacks such standardisation.
e) Acquisition: Colloquial Arabic is acquired naturally as a mother tongue, whereas standard Arabic is thought to be acquired later through formal schooling. However, Harry (1996) considered that these two varieties as a continuum rather than two distinct and separate language varieties, with classical Arabic at one end and vernacular Arabic at the other.

## 2 Dialectal Varieties of Arabic Language

Arabic is one of the six official languages of the United Nations (UN) and the most widely spoken language amongst the Semitic language family, and the fifth most spoken language globally. It is spoken by about 422 million both as a first and second language in the Arab world and other countries in Asia and Africa.

The regional Arabic dialects can be classified into six groups according to the levels of intelligibility as follows:

- Arabian Peninsula Arabic, spoken in Gulf countries and Yemen.
- Mesopotamian Arabic, spoken in Iraq.
- Levantine Arabic dialects, spoken in Lebanon, Syria, Jordan, and Palestine.
- Egyptian Arabic, the most spoken dialect and popular due to intensive use in the media, and to the fact that Egypt is by far the most populated country in the Arab world.
- Maghreb dialects, spoken in Morocco, Algeria, Tunisia, Libya and Mauritania.
- Sudanese Arabic, Spoken in Sudan and partially in Eritrea, Chad and Somalia.

The level of mutual intelligibility between the different regional dialects varies according to the geographical distance. However, based on particular linguistic features and clarity, some researchers (e.g., Maamouri, 1998) classified the regional Arabic dialects into two major geographical groups namely the Eastern dialects that are spoken in Morocco, Algeria, Tunisia, Libya and Mauritania, and Western dialects which are spoken in the rest of the Arab world.

## 3 Arabic Orthography and Diglossia

The orthography and writing system of Arabic language is an alphabetic cursive script that runs from right to left as opposed to Latin script. There are twenty-eight basic consonant letters in the alphabet, however, due to the cursive nature of the script twenty-two of the letters might have different shapes according to their position in the word, and thus they differ in initial, middle, final, or isolated positions (Bishop, 1999). Some consonant letters are identical in form and as such are distinguished from each other with additional diacritical dots or strokes. Additionally, diacritical forms are used for vocalic representations of short vowels and lexical differentiation. For instance, the base form of a word such as "KTBT" has five readings and five corresponding semantic interpretations: (a) *katabtu*: I wrote; (b) *katabta*: you (singular/masculine) wrote; (c) *katabti*: you (singular/feminine) wrote; (d) *katabat*: she wrote; and (e) *kutibat*: it (singular/feminine) was written.

Nevertheless, these short vowels are rarely used in everyday writing, and almost absent in printed materials, except in some cases such as in Quran or learning materials and books for the first stages of primary schools. In this regard, Abu-Rabia (1998) investigated the effect of vowels on reading accuracy in Arabic orthography. The most important finding of his study was that vowels were found to influence the reading of both poor and skilled readers significantly. It was also found that both skilled and poor readers improved their reading accuracy in all writing styles when they read with vowels. Hence, the Arabic orthographic system poses some challenges in the Arabic literacy domain as reflected in inefficient reading comprehension among Arab learners.

## 4 Impact of Diglossia on Literacy and Reading in Arabic

Literacy attainment, which is defined as the acquisition of a sustainable level of reading ability as a problematic area in the Arab world, since that literacy acquisition is by essence entails language acquisition and as such the diglossic nature of Arabic language seems to affect literacy attainment among Arab learners negatively. There is a clear consensus in the literature that the differences between classical and colloquial Arabic manifest themselves in all language domains (Holes, 1995). According to (Maamouri, 1998), all Arab educational systems suffer from high repetition and dropout rates. Also, illiteracy rates in the Arab world are higher than the average for developing countries and constitute a challenge for educational development.

Reading in Arabic seems to be a reversed process in which one first needs to understand to read, contrary to the usual norm in most other scripts and languages of the world, in which children or learners simply read to understand. Thus, language comprehension is seen as a pre-requisite to the acquisition of optimal reading skill in Arabic. This reading difficulty stems from the lack of vocalic representation within the Arabic writing system. For instance, it would be significantly difficult to read or interpret the meaning even of some single words, such as "دين/din", which might mean religion or debt according to the additional vocalic representations. They are mostly not written and have to be estimated in order to read or understand the word correctly by getting clues from the context in which the word is used. Similarly, Wagner (1993) indicated that there is a substantial reason to believe that learning to read in Arabic necessitates an even greater reliance on decoding skills than in other languages.

Moreover, children and even adult Arab readers cannot transfer their basic native linguistic competence in colloquial Arabic into the standard one. In this regard, Perfetti (1985) points out that the linguistic relatedness which exists between modern standard Arabic and the colloquial does not always provide helpful clues and does not necessarily contribute positively to successful reading defined merely as easy and fluid word recognition and language comprehension.

According to Maamouri (1998), Arabs, even highly educated ones, find it difficult and unnatural to use classical Arabic spontaneously without referring to a prepared text which is then partially or entirely read, and that Arab children are less able to read and write in classical or modern standard Arabic. The gap between standard Arabic as a language of formal education and the spoken dialect seemed to be a potential cause of the lower learning achievement and attained literacy rate among Arab children.

This inherent difficulty in Arabic reading comprehension led many researchers to claim that standard literary Arabic can be considered as a second language even for Arab speakers (Ayari, 1996; Eviatar & Ibrahim, 2000). For instance, Ibrahim (2009) suggests that the lexicon of literary Arabic is consistent with the typical organization of L2 in a separate lexicon. Thus, learning literary Arabic appears to be, in some respects, more like learning a second language than like learning the formal register of one's native language. In another empirical investigation, Ibrahim and Aharon-Peretz (2005) further concludes that despite the intensive daily use adult native Arabic speakers make of Spoken Arabic and literary Arabic, and despite their shared origin, the two languages retain their status as first and second languages in the cognitive system. Moreover, Eviatar and Ibrahim (2000) concluded that exposure to literary Arabic requires the same intensive language analyzes as those demanded of children exposed to languages as different as Russian and Hebrew.

# 5 Concluding Remarks

Arabic is usually thought of as one of the most diglossic languages with two distinct varieties switching from one language variety to another within the Arabic diglossic continuum to serve different functions. The lack of short vowels representation in the alphabet is idiosyncratic to Arabic, in addition to its cursive complex script that further influences the attainment of basic literacy skills among young and adult Arab learners alike.

Some researchers considered literary Arabic as a second language even for Arab speakers, and as such Arabic is no one mother tongue nowadays. This claim is based on some recent empirical psycholinguistic investigations, however, Parkinson (1991) argues that literary Arabic may not have native speakers, but it certainly has native users, people who read it fluently and listen to it with ease and understanding every day, and who occasionally use it in speaking and writing as well.

The effects of early exposure to Arabic literary texts on reading comprehension abilities are underestimated in the pre-schooling educational systems in the Arab world. Though, Abu-Rabia (2000) compared the reading comprehension performance of first and second-grade children who had been experimentally exposed to literary Arabic throughout their pre-schooling period with the reading performance of a parallel control group only exposed to spoken Arabic during that period. Contrary to the commonly held belief, the study found that the early exposure of Arab pre-school children to literary text and stories enhances their reading comprehension abilities and improves their performance in reading comprehension tests two years later.

Nevertheless, the high illiteracy rates of parents in the Arab world with some considerable regional variations, are disadvantageous for Arab children in attaining optimal basic literacy skills during the early pre-schooling years, which are quite critical for later and further literacy acquisition and in turn for their overall academic achievement in subsequent formal schooling stages. Moreover, a reconciliation between the high and low variety is also proposed to overcome the dilemma of the diglossic nature of Arabic. In this context, Wahba (2006) recommended teaching literacy and modern standard Arabic alongside a spoken colloquial variety of Arabic.

## 6 Affiliation

Dr. Adil Ishag
Institution: Faculty of Education, International University of Africa, Sudan.
Address: Madani St, Al Khurtum 12223, Sudan.
E-mail: adil.ishag@gmail.com

## 7 References

Abu-Rabia, S. (1998). Reading Arabic Texts: Effects of Text Type, Reader Type and Vowelization. *Reading and Writing: An Interdisciplinary Journal, 10*, 105–119.

Abu-Rabia, S. (2000). Effects of Exposure to Literary Arabic on Reading Comprehension in a Diglossic Situation. *Reading and Writing: An Interdisciplinary Journal, 13*, 147–157.

Ayari, S. (1996). Diglossia and Illiteracy in the Arab World. *Language, Culture and Curriculum, 9*, 243–252.

Bishop, R. (1999). *A history of the Arabic Language.* Salt Lake City, UT: Brigham Young University.

Eviatar, Z., & Ibrahim, R. (2000). Bilingual is as Bilingual Does: Metalinguistic Abilities of Arabic-speaking Children. *Applied Psycholinguistics, 21*(4), 451–471.

Ferguson, C. A. (1959). Diglossia. *Word, 15*(2), 325–340.

Fishman, J. A. (1970). *Sociolinguistics: A Brief Introduction.* Rowley: Newbury House Publishers.

Hary, B. (1996). The Importance of the Language Continuum in Arabic Multiglossia." In A. Elgibali (Ed.), *Understanding Arabic: Essays in Contemporary Arabic Linguistics in Honor of El-Said Badawi* (pp.66–90). Cairo: The American University in Cairo Press.

Holes, C. (1995). *Modern Arabic: Structures, Functions, and Varieties.* London: Longman.

Ibrahim, R., & Aharon-Peretz, J. (2005). Is literacy Arabic a second language for native Arab speakers?: Evidence from semantic priming study. *Journal of Psycholinguistic Research, 34*(1), 51–70.

Ibrahim, R. (2009). The Cognitive Basis of Diglossia in Arabic: Evidence from a Repetition Priming Study within and Between Languages. *Psychology Research and Behavior Management, 2*, 93–105.

Maamouri, M. (1998). *Language Education and Human Development: Arabic Diglossia and its Impact on the Quality of Education in the Arab Region.* Discussion Paper Prepared for The World Bank Mediterranean Development Forum, Marrakesh. Philadelphia: University of Pennsylvania International Literacy Institute.

Palmer, J. (2007). Arabic Diglossia: Teaching Only the Standard Variety is a Disservice to Students. *Arizona Working Papers in SLA & Teaching, 14*, 111–122.

Parkinson, D. B. (1991). Searching for Modern *fusha*: Real-life Formal Arabic. *Al-Arabiyya, 24*, 31–64.

Perfetti, C. A. (1985). *Reading Ability.* New York: Oxford University Press.

Wagner, D. A. (1993). *Literacy, Culture, and Development: Becoming Literate in Morocco.* Cambridge: Cambridge University Press.

Wahba, K. M. (2006). Arabic Language Use and the Educated Language User. In K. M. Wahba, Z. A. Taha, & L. England (Eds.), *Handbook for Arabic Language Teaching Professionals* (pp. 139–155). Mahwah, NJ: Lawrence Erlbaum.

Raziq Ouafa

# Die Bedeutsamkeit des Phänomens Legasthenie in Marokko

**Abstract:** Participation in social, cultural, political and economic life requires reading and writing. In order to obtain a minimum education, it is important for every person to learn to read, write and calculate in primary school. Early detection of problems in writing and reading the pupil already in elementary school is important to develop appropriate intervention programs for treatment. The aim of this paper is to use an interview with teachers in two different types of schools in Casablanca to verify that they have the knowledge and expertise to do dyslexia. It would also be important to know what measures are taken if they find these cases in their school and to what extent the Ministry of Education takes account of the problem.

**Keywords:** reading and spelling weakness, reading and writing skills, dyslexia, problems of the Arabic script

**Zusammenfassung:** Die Teilnahme am gesellschaftlichen, kulturellen, politischen und wirtschaftlichen Leben erfordert das Lesen und Schreiben. Zum Erwerb einer minimalen Ausbildung, ist es für jeden Menschen wichtig, das Lesen, Schreiben und Rechnen in der Grundschule zu lernen. Eine Früherkennung von Problemen beim Schreiben und Lesen des Schülers bereits in der Grundschule ist bedeutend, um passende Interventionsprogramme für die Behandlung zu entwickeln. Ziel dieser Arbeit ist es, anhand eines Interviews mit Lehrern in zwei verschiedenen Schularten in Casablanca zu überprüfen, ob diese über Kenntnisse und Wissen, in Hinblick auf Legasthenie verfügen. Wichtig wäre auch zu wissen, welche Maßnahmen getroffen werden, falls sie in ihrer Schule diese Fälle vorfinden und inwieweit das Bildungsministerium Rücksicht auf das Problem nimmt.

**Schlussworte:** Lese- und Rechtschreibschwäche, Lese- und Rechtschreibfertigkeiten, Legasthenie, Probleme der Arabischen Schrift

## 1 Einleitung

Probleme beim Erwerb von schulischen Fertigkeiten des Lesens und Schreibens sind relativ häufig vorkommende, umschriebene Entwicklungsstörungen, die in allen Schriftsprachen beobachtet werden. Die Lese- und Schreibkompetenz spielt eine bedeutsame Rolle für jeden Menschen, sowohl im Privatleben als auch in der Gesellschaft, in der Schule und im Arbeitsbereich, vom aktiven Engagement am gesellschaftlichen Leben bis hin zum lebenslangen Lernen. Lesen und schreiben zu können ist ein Grundprinzip und eine Grundanforderung jeder Gesellschaft.

Wenn jemand unter Lese- und Rechtschreibschwäche leidet, besteht die Gefahr, ins Abseits gedrängt zu werden. Darüber schreibt Füssenich (1999, S. 183). „Wer in der Schule lese-und rechtschreibschwach ist und bleibt, wird nach der Schulentlassung zu den funktionalen Analphabeten/innen gehören".

Um das Problem zu beseitigen, ist es erforderlich eine Frühfeststellung von Mängeln der Schüler/innen bei den Lese- Rechtschreibfertigkeiten zu erkennen, um entsprechende Förder- und Interventionsprogramme für die Behandlung zu entwickeln. Man vermutet, dass ungefähr 10% der Weltbevölkerung von der Legasthenie betroffen sind. Man schätzt, dass etwa 8 % von Kindern in Marokko von Legasthenie betroffen sind.

In Marokko war es schwer exakte Angaben über Legasthenie zu erhalten, da selbst Pädagogen nur über geringe Informationen zum Störungsbild verfügen. Man muss darauf verweisen, dass die ökonomischen, sozialen und kulturellen Faktoren als Ursachenerklärungen für die mangelnde Schriftsprachkompetenz in Marokko und Deutschland eine grundlegende Rolle spielen (Raziq, 2006).

Anhand eines Interviews mit Lehrern in zwei unterschiedlichen staatlichen und privaten Schulen in Casablanca wollen wir wissen, ob sich Lehrer überhaupt mit dem Phänomen „Dyslexie" auskennen und ob es Kinder mit Lese-Rechtschreibschwierigkeiten gibt. Zu prüfen wäre, welche Fördermaßnahmen angeboten werden, falls dieses Problem erkannt wird und inwieweit das Bildungsministerium Rücksicht darauf nimmt und Interventionsmöglichkeiten anbietet.

## 2 Charakteristik der Arabischen Sprache

Das Arabische wird in Hochsprache und Dialekte bzw. Umgangssprache gegliedert. Das Arabische gehört bekanntlich zu den semitischen Sprachen. Geschrieben wird das Arabische von rechts nach links auf der Grundlage des arabischen Alphabets, das nur Konsonanten und Langvokale kennt.

In phonetischer Hinsicht ist die arabische Sprache dadurch charakterisiert, dass die Vokale nicht geschrieben werden. Was dazu führen kann, dass Wörter gleich geschrieben werden, aber verschieden gesprochen werden, z. B. KTB. Dieses aus 3 Konsonanten ohne Vokale geschriebene Wort kann in verschiedenen Varianten gesprochen werden (*Kataba, Kotiba, Kotobon*), was zwangsläufig zu verschiedenen Bedeutungen führt und deshalb die Lernenden irritiert und verwirrt und damit Schreibfehler verursacht werden. Das gilt vor allem für die Kurzvokale A, I und U sowie für die Konsonantenverdopplung. Für Legastheniker bietet diese Besonderheit der arabischen Schrift eine starke Erschwernis beim Erlernen der Schriftsprache.

Diese Erscheinung gilt besonders für die arabische Schriftsprache, in der die Vokale fehlen. Besonders Kinder im Schulalter leiden darunter, wenn sie beginnen das Lesen und Schreiben zu lernen.

Deswegen bedienen sich die Lehrer in den Volksschulen der Methode der so genannten „Vokalzeichen" (*Chakl*). Für Lernanfänger des Arabischen werden die Kurzvokale geschrieben, weil sie eine entscheidende Rolle im Erlernen des Lesens und Rechtschreibens spielen (Abu-Rabia, 2002). Weiterhin haben sie eine zusätzliche Rolle hinsichtlich der Identifizierung der grammatikalischen Funktion der Wörter in den Sätzen, welche auf syntaktischen Kenntnissen basieren (Abu-Rabia, 2002).

## 3 Das Schul- und Bildungssystem in Marokko

Viele marokkanische Eltern misstrauen dem staatlichen Schulsystem. In den Städten hat das kostenlose staatliche Schulsystem einen miserablen Ruf. Wer es sich leisten kann, schickt seine Kinder auf Privatschulen. Dadurch entsteht in Marokko eine Zwei-Klassen-Bildungsgesellschaft. Heute zu berichten über das marokkanische Schulsystem, heißt den Blick auf die Gesamtbevölkerung zu werfen.

Angesicht der wirtschaftlichen Lage des Landes lebt ein großer Teil der Bevölkerung in Armut. So können viele Familien zwar ihre Kinder in die Schule schicken, jedoch müssen die Kinder die Schule frühzeitig verlassen, da die Schulen sowie die Kinder von dem Staat nicht genügend unterstützt werden. In den meisten Schulen findet man schlechte Bedingungen: Die Schülerzahl in der Klasse ist enorm, etwa 50 Schüler in der Klasse, meistens schlechte Schüler-Lehrer-Beziehungen bzw. Interaktionen und das Personal ist nicht fortgebildet, um eine ordentliche Leistung zu gewährleisten.

Schüler aus armen Familien sind hinsichtlich der materiellen Ausstattung (z.B. Schulbücher) sowie hinsichtlich der Zeit, die für das Lernen aufgebracht werden kann, erheblich benachteiligt. Viele Kinder werden von ihren Eltern dazu bewogen, ihre Schule zu unterbrechen, damit sie eventuell zum Unterhalt der Familie beitragen können. Nur ein geringer wohlhabender Teil der Marokkaner ist in der Lage, seine Kinder auf private Schulen zu schicken.

Nach offiziellen Angaben wurden jedoch seit Beginn des Schuljahres 1998/99 ebenso viele Mädchen wie Jungen eingeschult. Die Schulpflicht gilt für Kinder im Alter von 7 bis 13 Jahren.

## 4 Zum Begriff Legasthenie

Charakteristisch für die Lese-Rechtschreibschwäche (LRS) ist der Umstand, dass die Betroffenen Leserechtschreibfähigkeiten verzögert und erschwert erwerben. Diese Probleme können nicht auf alternative Ursachen zurückgeführt werden, wie mangelhafte Beschulung, emotionale bzw. neurologische Störungen und Intelligenzminderung.

Das Problem des Schriftspracherwerbes wurde zum ersten Mal am Ende des 19. Jahrhundert erörtert. Der Begriff Legasthenie wurde von dem ungarischen Neurologen Paul Ranschburg (1916) gebraucht (in Warnke, 1990). Ranschburg sprach zum ersten Mal vom Aspekt phonologischer Defizite, indem er nicht nur auf visuelle Verwechselungs-fehler, sondern auch auf solche phonologischer Art bezogen auf ähnliche Laute hinwies. Maria Lindner (1951) definierte Legasthenie als Teilleistungsstörung, indem sie sich auf die Gedanken von Morgans stützte. Seitdem findet das Phänomen Legasthenie seinen Platz in der wissenschaftlichen Forschung. Es gibt unterschiedliche Definitionen zum Terminus Legasthenie. So reichen die verwendeten Begriffe von Störung der Schriftsprache (u.a. Berkhan, 1885; Ranschburg, 1916) bis zu entwicklungsbedingter Lesestörung (Warnke, 1990).

In anderen Ländern spricht man von Dyslexia. Auch im arabischen Sprachraum gibt es Definitionen, die sich nicht von denen aus England und Frankreich unterscheiden. In einer Studie schreibt Alhamdan (1992) (in Taha, 2002), dass die Leseschwäche in der arabischen Sprache durch folgende Kriterien charakterisiert ist:

- Mangel an Grundlagen des Lesens, was auch die Fächer betrifft, die nicht direkt das Lesen zum Gegenstand haben wie Geometrie und Mathematik.
- Die Unfähigkeit, zwischen den verschiedenen Buchstaben zu unterscheiden.
- Vernachlässigung und Weglassen wichtiger, grundlegender Bestandteile des Schreibens wie Punkte und Verwechslung ähnlicher Buchstabenformen (س=S) (س=s: stimmloser dentaler Reibelaut) und (ش=sch) (ش=š: stimmloser palato-alveolar).

# 5 Methode

Im Rahmen einer wissenschaftlichen Studie haben wir ein Interview mit Lehrern aus verschiedenen Institutionen in Casablanca geführt, um zu sehen, ob Lehrer sich überhaupt mit dem Legasthenie Phänomen auskennen und wie sie damit umgehen. An diesem Interview nahmen 20 Lehrer und Lehrerinnen aus staatlichen und privaten Schulen teil.

# 6 Ergebnisse

Die Ergebnisse dieser Studie ergaben, dass die Mehrheit der befragten Lehrer, welche in privaten Schulen eingestellt sind, mit dem Legasthenie Phänomen vertraut sind. Die Lehrer aus öffentlichen Schulen haben wenig oder überhaupt keine Ahnung, was mit der Legasthenie gemeint ist. Die Lehrer aus beiden Schulen können nichts unternehmen, da die Schule keine Achtung und Aufmerksamkeit für solche Kinder hat. Weiterhin berichten sie, dass diese Kinder mit den anderen Mitschülern, die überhaupt keine Lese- und Rechtschreibprobleme haben, zusammengemischt sind, obwohl sie Förderunterricht dringend und frühzeitig benötigen. Zukünftig hoffen die Lehrer auf eine Aus- und Fortbildung betreffend des Themas Legasthenie. Die Lehrer aus beiden Schularten behaupten, dass ihre Institutionen über keine Instrumente verfügen, welche sie beim Umgang mit den betroffenen Kindern nutzen können. Sie bestätigen, dass das Schulbildungsministerium nicht in irgendeiner Weise interveniert bezüglich der Schwierigkeiten von Schülern im Lesen und Schreiben. Sie behaupten auch, dass das Ministerium keine Rücksicht auf diese Problematik nimmt und auch keine pädagogischen und didaktischen Methoden für diese Schülern anbietet, um das Problem zu mindern. Das Ministerium bietet auch keine spezielle Ausbildung für Lehrer, um eine wirksame Begleitung dieser Kinder zu erreichen.

Weiterhin behaupten die Lehrer, dass durch das Ministerium keine spezielle Förderung bei Schreib- und Leseschwierigkeiten als auch keine speziellen Klassen für solche Kinder zu Verfügung gestellt werden. Die Lehrer hoffen, dass das Schulbildungsministerium pädagogische Programme im Rahmen der gesamten akademischen Schullaufbahn entwickelt und zur Verfügung stellt.

Da die Problematik der Lese-Rechtschreibschwäche kaum Beachtung in der arabischen Welt erfährt, existieren auch keine wissenschaftlich fundierten psychodiagnostischen Testverfahren. So sind Legastheniker trotz normaler Intelligenz und normalen Hörens konfrontiert mit Misserfolg wegen ihrer extremen Schwierigkeiten, geschriebene Wörter zu erkennen. Es ist wichtig zu betonen, dass sich die Vorstellung und Diagnostik in Schulen als eine Notwendigkeit für die normale Entwicklung und die Gesundheit des Kindes erforderlich erweist (Ahami et al., 2006; Badda et al., 2008).

## 7 Diskussion

Die Beherrschung des Lesens und Schreibens ist zu einer Schlüsselkompetenz in jeder Gesellschaft geworden, in welcher der Schul- und Berufserfolg als auch die sozialen Entwicklungschancen davon abhängig sind. In unserer marokkanischen Gesellschaft als auch in der Schule wird Legasthenie noch immer mit Dummheit, Unkonzentriertheit und Faulheit verwechselt. Daher muss man sagen, dass das Wissen um das Phänomen Legasthenie leider nur gering ausgeprägt ist. Das Marokkanische Schulbildungssystem erkennt die Existenz dieser kognitiven Störung nicht an. Aber einige Publikationen in Marokko weisen indirekt auf das Phänomen der „Legasthenie" bei den Kindern auf der Schulebene sowohl auch in der arabischen Sprache als auch in der französischen Sprache als zweiter Fremdsprache hin (Badda, 2008). Es gibt keine klare und logische Interpretation von Seiten der meisten Lehrer betreffend dieses Problems der Lese- und Rechtschreibschwierigkeiten. Selbst Pädagogen verfügen über keine Kenntnisse hinsichtlich dieser Problematik.

## 8 Affiliation

Dr. Ouafa Raziq
Institution: Université Hassan II, Ain Chok
Address: 17 Rue Amyot, Quartier des Hôpitaux, App 5 Casablanca Marokko
E-mail: ouafaeadam@hotmail.fr

## 9 Referenzliste

Abu-Rabia, S. (2002). Reading in a root-based morphology language. *Journal of Research in Reading, 25,* 299–309.

Ahami, A. O. T., Mari, E., Aboussalah, Y., Biyadi, N., Azzaoui, F. Z., Samih, M., Mesfioui, A., & Elbouhali, B. (2006). Dépistage des troubles psychomoteurs et comportementaux chez le jeune enfant. *Santé, Education et Environnement,* 33–41. Rabat: Digi Edition.

Badda, B. (2008). *Apprentissage de la lecture, dyslexie phonologique et remédiation par lelogiciel « Itinéraire Combinatoire » chez l'enfant marocain.* (Unpublished Doctoral Dissertation). Université Ibn Tofail, Cotutelle – Université de Rennes 2, France.

Badda, B., Ahami, A. O. T., Aboussaleh, Y., Bahtit, J., & Gombert, J. E. (2008). Repérage des difficultés d'apprentissage de lecture évoquant la dyslexie phonologique chez des enfants marocains. *Pathologies Humaines et Déficits de Développement Approche Pluridisciplinaire.* Edition Imprimerie Rapide, 33–37.

Berkhan, O. (1885). Über die Schriftsprache bei Halbidioten und ihre Ähnlichkeit mit dem Stammeln. *Archiv für Psychiatrie, 16,* 78–86.

Füssenich, I. (1999). *Funktionaler Analphabetismus in Deutschland.* In Gombert, J. E., Colé, P., Valdois, S., Goigoux, R., Mousty, P., & Fayol, M. (Eds.), *Enseigner la lecture au cycle 2,* (pp.183–188). Paris: Nathan Pédagogie.

Lindner, M. (1951). Über Legasthenie (spezielle Leseschwäche). *Zeitschrift für Kinder-Psychiatrie, 17,* 97.

Ranschburg. (1916). *Die Leseschwäche (Legasthenie) und Rechenschwäche (Arithmasthenie) der Schulkinder im Licht des Experimentes.* Berlin: Springer.

Raziq, O. (2006). *Verteilung der sozioökonomischen Status von Legasthenikern und Normallesenden.* Unpulished Manuscript.

Taha, D. (2002). *Schwierigkeiten beim Lesen und Schreiben der arabischen Sprachebei bilingualen Schuelern.* (Unpublished Master Thesis). Alchams University, Cairo, Ägypten.

Warnke, A. (1990). *Legasthenie und Hirnfunktion: Neuropsychologische Befunde zur visuellen Informationsverarbeitung.* Bern: Verlag Hans Huber.

Khaled Youssef Alammar

# A Study of Dyslexia among Fourth Class Pupils in Rural Daraa according to Some Variables

**Abstract:** This research aimed to the study of dyslexia among forth class pupils in rural Daraa according to some variables. This study was donewitha clear analytic method. The intended sample was pupils ($n = 200$) from forth class pupils in rural Daraa. Dyslexia Scale (DS) was built in this study according to methical steps which are used in a scale structure. The results showed the followings: The distribution is normal, there is negative relationship between dyslexia and academic level of parents (-0.20), but there is no relationship between dyslexia and numbers of failure years, the boys have dyslexia more than girls.

**Keywords:** dyslexia, fourth class pupils in rural Daraa, Dyslexia Scale

## 1 Introduction

The theoretical concept of dyslexia is to be clarified. This term has two-fold, "dys" means weakness or difficulty, and "lexia" means words or vocabulary (Batayneh, 2005). The prevalence of dyslexia among students is 10%, and males are more than females. Every four males are matched by one female. Some studies have reported that seven males vs one female (Sheikh Hamoud & Alammar, 2012). Dyslexia was explained in light of several theoretical trends. The first trend was that they were due to brain damage or malfunction. The second trend is the abnormal growth of some brain cells, through physiological studies indicating that there is an abnormal increase in the number of neurons in the nerve centres of the brain. The third trend is the genetic trend, which indicates that dyslexia is due to hereditary factors (Btatya & Bukasi, 2013). As for the symptoms of dyslexia, for example mixing in order such as days, months, letters, etc., improper pronunciation, incorrect writing, incorrect spelling, errors in directions, reverse of similar letters memory and forgetfulness, introversion, difficulty in languages and mathematics, letter confusion, poor concentration, inaccuracy of writing, reading of words or numbers conversely, or excessive slowness with inconsistency, fear and mistrust, dizziness, sweating, vomiting, dyspepsia, etc. (Vernon, 1976). The causes of dyslexia are tension in the family or school, fear, neglect, loss of trust and sympathetic understanding (Newton, Thomson, & Richards, 1984). Educational reasons are also explained, such as learning methods and methods of negative dealing with the school (Rutter & Yule, 1975). Critchley's educational reasons for educational purposes related to general education conditions and programscauses related to the goals of the reading and assessment program, and reasons for poor teaching methods (Critchley & Critchley, 1978). Neuropathy and neurotoxicity are also associated with the visual system (Vellutino, 1980). Pugh et al., (2001) add that the problem is related to brain dysfunction, which is double the storage and retrieval of memory (Pugh et al., 2001). Also, previously Galaburda, Sherman, Rosen, Aboitiz, and Geschwind (1985) found that the brain of the disabled has two types of anatomical anomalies affecting the ability to read and write. Genetic causes through the study of genes for the disabled and their families have confirmed that there is a genetic defect that proves that dyslexia is genetic, and this has also been demonstrated by surveys (Stein & Glenn, 1996).

## 2 Research Problem

The research problem emerged through two primary sources: personal observations first and the previous literature. It has been noted that a few students have great difficulty or difficulty in learning English. When being asked by some teachers in English about the reality of these observations, it was confirmed by them. Teachers have included a number of observations, such as difficulties to pronounce the word correctly, headache, dizziness and physical complaint, change of characters while typing or numbers, redness of the face during reading, lack of punctuation, confusion in the order of days or months, difficulty in identifying and selecting from a multiple-answer question, suffering from shyness and confusion when reading and writing, increase characters of difficulty, the lack of self-confidence even if the correct answer is known, sweating while reading, fear while in class, forgetfulness, difficulty of remembering the spelling rules, difficulty in memorizing similar words and other observations made by teachers about these students.

These realistic observations have been a driving force for research, stimulating motivation for research into dyslexia. The first source (personal notes) has also led to research in previous literature on the subject of dyslexia, whether in Arabic or foreign studies. It is noted that the Arab and international studies have confirmed the existence of difficulty in reading and writing among some students, which necessitated research on this subject. From here, the problem of research can be summed up by the following question: What is the nature of dyslexia according to a range of demographic variables such as the educational level of parents and the number of years of repetition and gender?

## 3 Research Aims

This study of dyslexia among the fourth-grade students in the elementary schools of rural Daraa aims to measure dyslexia according to some demographic variables and examining the differences between students in dyslexia according to the gender variable.

## 4 Research Questions

1) What is the nature of the distribution of dyslexia?
2) What are the differences in dyslexia among students in light of demographic variables such as the educational level of parents, the number of years of repetition andgender?

## 5 Research Hypotheses

1) There is no statistically significant relationship between dyslexia and the educational level of parents.
2) There is no statistically significant relationship between dyslexia and the number of years of repetition.
3) There is a statistically significant difference in dyslexia due to the gender factor.

## 6 Theoretical Review

Radwan's study (1992) explains a program to reduce dyslexia in mathematics among students in the fourth grade of elementary school in Egypt. The results show that there is a difference between the experimental group and the control group. It is due to the effectiveness of the program in reducing dyslexia and mathematics among the fourth-grade students in primary education. Based on Bashir's Study (2006), the reflection of dyslexia on the aggressive behavior of Al-Misorin in Algeriahave shown that there is a positive correlation between dyslexia and aggressive behavior among students.

Meanwhile, Btatya and Boukasi (2013) on their study of the relationship of hyperactivity with Attention Deficit in the appearance of dyslexia in fourth-year primary students conducted a field study of seven cases in Algeria. The results show that there was a positive correlation between hyperactivity with attention deficit and dyslexia among fourth-year primary students. Also, Hashani and Nawar (2016) study psychological and orthopaedic guarantees for dyslexia of fourth-year students in Algeria. The results show that the psychological and orthopaedic bonding program is highly effective in reducing dyslexia on the sample.

Further, from west literature, Butler (as cited in Saidi, 2009) in his study of the effect of an integrated and innovative reading therapy program using the multi-branch readymade training package in an advanced classification show that there is a difference in favour of the experimental group on the control. The application was repeated on the fifth-grade students. The result was also in favour of the pilot (Butler as cited in Saidi, 2009). Also, in the study of Mathers and Fuchs (as cited in Saidi, 2009) about the effect of using recurrent reading methods and reading support method, the results prove the effectiveness in both ways of treating dyslexia (Mathers and Fuchs as cited in Saidi, 2009). Research from Tanner (2009) about adult dyslexia and "The Failure Puzzle" in Australia show there are several forms of failure experienced by the disabled. They are 1) the failure of the educational system to deal with this category, 2) the failure to discriminate in the laws against the disabled and indirectly deal with them as disabled, 3) the general failure is determined by the behavior of colleagues and others towards the disabled, with impotence and reflection on it, which may lead the personal failure of the insolvent to suicidal thoughts. Later, Łodygowska and Czepita (2012) in their study offear of school in children with dyslexia show that dyslexics females suffer from school fear more than dyslexic males, as well as related treatment methods, contribute to reducing the fear of the disabled, unlike the irregular or traditional ways.

# 7 Method

Method of search limits was done to some towns and cities including Daraa, where the schools are located in the first ring of primary education, which includes fourth-grade students. This research was conducted in early 2017. The field research was appliedat the end of the second semester in the academic year 2017–2018.

# 8 Terms and Procedural Definitions

Dyslexia, according to the British Society for Literacy defines as "a particular difficulty in learning that hinders the learning of basic skills in reading, writing, spelling, and mathematics. This problem is in dealing with verbal codes in memory, andits basis is nervous and tends to be inherited in families, which can be at any level of intelligence, and the effects of dyslexia can be reduced by teaching by teachers trained in modern teaching methods" (Saidi, 2009, p. 28–29). As defined by the International Association of Dyslexia, dyslexia is "a disorder that has – often – agenetic origin, and makes it difficult to learn and address the language in a listening and expression, and includes problems in speech, reading, writing, spelling and handwriting and sometimes in mathematics" (Karima, 2016, p. 218).

The procedural definition of dyslexia is defined as the degree to which the subject is obtained on the scale of dyslexia that was built in this research. This degree starts after the first deviation in the positive direction by 1.01 (Z-score).

The educational level of the parents represents the certificate carried by the parents. The educational level in the research was given four levels as follows: elementary = 1, preparatory = 2, secondary = 3, above secondary school or university = 4.

## 8.1 Design of the Research and Determine its Procedural Steps on Research Methodology

The descriptive analytical method was adopted in this research, which is defined as "one of the forms of analysis and scientific interpretation that is organized to describe the phenomenon or the specific problem and quantify it by collecting data and information disaggregated on the phenomenon or problem" (Melhem, 2000,

**Table 1.** Total number of students regarding sex (male, female) and sample

| Number of students | | Number of samples | Percentage of total number |
|---|---|---|---|
| Males | 7,951 | 100 | 1.257% |
| Females | 7,870 | 100 | 1.270% |
| Total | 15,821 | 200 | 1.264% |

p. 324). According to this method, information was collected through research tools, namely, the measure of dyslexia and writing, and then the raw data was emptied through SPSS 22 statistical program. This information was analyzed quantitatively through a set of laws and tests that are tested questions and hypotheses. The results were interpreted in light of the theoretical aspect and the specificity of the environment and culture of the research society. The results were also discussed in comparison to previous studies, whether Arab or foreign. The points of agreement and disagreement were shown and explanations of this difference if any.

## 8.2 Research Community and Sample

The research community is a fourth-grade student in the elementary schools in the rural governorate of Daraa, the number of pupils in the fourth grade, according to the official records at the Directorate of Education in Daraa are 15,821 students. The sample of the research was 200 students, which consisted of 100 males and 100 females as well, and the sample was deliberately drawn from the schools of rural Daraa. The sample is based on the researcher's experience and knowledge to get students who have dyslexia. The chosen sample represents the research community well served, for example when the researcher selects a group of schools; he is tortured. It is the responsibility of the researcher to use these types of samples to justify the scientific justification, so as not to be accused of bias (Alammar, 2014). The research was applied in 13 schools.

## 8.3 Search Tools

The measure of dyslexia in this research has been built by the researcher according to methodological steps and can be summarised as follows:

1) Defining the concept of dyslexia and reading.
2) The definition of dyslexia is a practical or functional definition used on the field side and is defined as a measure of the degree to which the subject is obtained on the scale of reading and writing. This degree starts after the first deviation in the positive direction and by 1.01 standard score (Z-score).
3) Analysis of dyslexia. This analysis is a quantitative.
4) Determination of weights of factors.

5) Suggestion of items.
6) Survey Study. A survey was conducted on the scale in its initial form, through the application to 30 students and answered by the English teachers.
7) Application of the measure of dyslexia on the original sample was done after the previous steps were applied to the original sample measure of 200 students, but the answer to this measure are the English teachers, not the pupils.

### 8.4 Validity of the Measure

Validity of the measure, actually, is accomplished in several ways:

*8.4.1 The researches' validity*

The scale was presented to a group of English language teachers for the fourth-grade students. Ten teachers determine the validity of the measure. It is what is called the sincerity of the arbitrators. Allen and Yen (1979, p. 96) states: "The best way to extract virtual truth is to present the paragraphs of the scale to a group of arbitrators to judge their validity in measuring the property to be measured". The objective of the scale presentation was to verify the truth by the following points: The appropriateness of the measure to the purpose for which it was established, the integrity of the terms concerning language formulation, addition, deletion or modification of what was inappropriate from their point of view. After making the observations of the arbitrators, each item was kept or amended in which the proportion of the agreement between the arbitrators increased by 60% according to the Lawshe's method in this regard (Abdul Rahman, 2003). Five items were amended to meet the requirements of the fourth grade English course.

*8.4.2 Discriminatory of validity*

The highest quarter was taken from the sample regarding the level of grades (25%) and the lowest quarter (25%). Then the t-test was used. The result shows that the scale has a significant discriminant capacity.

*8.4.3 Factor analysis*

The analysis was carried out according to Principal Component Analysis method in the program (SPSS-22) that they are best in the division and analysis of the factors represented by dyslexia. The Matrix Component Matrix method leads to five factors: *Factor 1* = reading (13 items), *factor 2* = writing (13 items), *factor 3* = memory (11 items), *factor 4* = self-compatibility (16 items), *factor 5* = spelling (8 items). Extraction of all items was higher than 0.30.

Subjective validity is based on the coefficient of the stability of the scale by repetition, where it is the square root of the stability coefficient (Abdul Rahman,

2003). The stability by repetition is 0.89 at significant level ($p$) = 0.01. When calculating the square root of this stability to reach the self-confidence of the scale, it was found to be equal to 94.0. This is another indication of the validity of the scale to measure what was measured. The relationship values between different factors of dyslexia scale are about 0.66 and 0.20.

## 8.5 Reliability of the Scale

Achieved reliability in several ways is:

1) Reliability by re-stability: The test was re-applied three weeks after its application the first time. The re-application resulted in a Pearson correlation was 0.89 ($p$ = 0.01) and the number of sample were 50 students.
2) Reliability by dipping or retailing: The scale was divided into two halves where the first half included the individual items while the second half included the matrimonial items. The results showed a Pearson correlation between the two halves equal to 0.92 ($p$ = 0.01) and the sample were 200 students.
3) Reliability in internal consistency: The coefficient of Cronbach's alpha ($\alpha$ = 0.92).

The correlation of the scale factors was measured with the scale as a whole between 0.62 and 0.84.

## 8.6 Preparation of Standard Tables (Correction of the Dyslexia Scale)

The score of the subject was calculated and evaluated using the standard score or Z-score by descriptive statistics and the standard scores in SPSS-22. The results of the Kolmogorov-Smirnoff test (KS-test) to detect the distribution of the sample were 1.16 (non-significant) (14.0). It means that the sample has a normal distribution. The value of kurtosis is -0.15 which also indicated the normal distribution of the sample. The values are mostly around the average and gradually decrease in the direction of the limbs. It is noted that there is a tendency in the distribution towards the positive party, that is, the sample has dyslexia. As long as the distribution is normal, this means that the tests to be used in this study are parametric tests that are suitable for normal distribution.

# 9 Results

## 9.1 There is no statistically significant relationship between dyslexia and literacy and the educational level of parents

Pearson's correlation was used to determine the relationship between dyslexia and educational level of parents. The correlation value -0.20 was at a level of significance of 0.02. Therefore, there is a negative relationship between the variables.

This relationship is weak but functional. It means that the higher the parental certificate, the lower the dyslexia of students. It may be normal, as parents with high degrees transfer their experience in dealing with the study to boys, making them more compatible with the study requirements. The children learn from the parents the method of study and how to prepare for the exam; the method of writing duties and the way of thinking; and the search for sources to help the student understand books and networking and other sources of knowledge. All of this makes it easier for students to study requirements and falls in the field of compatibility. This result has not been found in previous studies to be compared with them.

## 9.2 There is no significant relationship between dyslexia and the number of years of repetition

This hypothesis was tested by Pearson's correlation to detect the relationship between dyslexia and the number of years of repetition. The correlation value 0.10 was not significant, which means that there is no correlation between the two variables. Dyslexia does not mean that a student with low intelligence and little achievement shows the impact of difficulty on achievement. The student is often insoluble as an intelligent child and not low intelligence, and maybe some insolvent geniuses. The most obvious is Albert Einstein, the theory of relativity, which was dyslexic. But dyslexia did not prevent him from excellence and creativity.

## 9.3 There is a significant difference in dyslexia due to gender

A t-test was used to study the differences to test this hypothesis. The results show that males have more dyslexia than females, thus believing the hypothesis. It may be due to the centre of language in the brain, which is characterized as more mature in females than males to adolescence. Studies indicate that the number of dyslexic males exceeds the number of females. This result is in line with the statements made by Sheikh Hamoud and Alammar (2012) that the prevalence of dyslexia among males is higher than that of females. Every four males are interviewed by one female. Some studies say that seven males versus one female.

# 10 Research Suggestions and Future Research

It is found the benefit from the scale that has been built in new research on dyslexia. The defining of the nature of dyslexia through a media awareness campaign addresses the characteristics of the dyslexic child and guides parents to deal with it. It is necessary to study new research linking dyslexia and new variables, including the construction of psychological programs to treat cases of dyslexia.

## 11 Affiliation

Dr. Khaled Yousef Alammar
Institution: Department of Psychological Counselling, Faculty of Education, Damascus University, Syria.
Address: Syria, Damascus, Bramka, Damascus University, Faculty of Education, Department of Psychological Counselling.
E-mail: omarkh72@hotmail.com

## 12 References

Abdul Rahman, S. (2003). *Psychometric measurement: Theory and practice, I, 4.* Cairo: Arab Thought House.

Alammar, K. Y. (2014). *Alphabetical research and preparation of academic messages in the psychological, educational and social sciences.* Amman: Scientific Alasar House for Publishing and Distribution.

Allen, M. J., & Yen, W. M. (1979). *Introduction to measurement theory.* Monterey, CA: Brooks/Cole.

Bashir, S. (2006). *The reflection of dyslexia on the aggressive behaviour of dyslexics.* Algeria: Collage of Social Sciences.

Batayneh, B. O. (2005). *Learning difficulties and theoretical practice, I.* Amman: Dar Al - Maysara for Publication and Distribution.

Btatya, Z. & Boukasi, F. (2013). *The relationship of hyperactivity with Attention Deficit in the appearance of dyslexia in fourth year primary students: A field study of seven cases from 6–9 years* (Unpublished Thesis). University of AkhalMohandOulhaj, Faculty of Social and Human Sciences, Algeria.

Critchley, M., & Critchley, E. R. (1978). *Dyslexia defined.* London: Heinemann Medical Books.

Galaburda, A. M., Sherman, G. F., Rosen, G. D., Aboitiz, F., & Geschwind, N. (1985). Developmental dyslexia: Four consecutive patients with cortical anomalies. *Annals of Neurology, 18,* 222–233.

Hashani, S., & Nawar, S. (2016). Psychological and orthodontic sponsorship for those who have difficulty writing from fourth year primary students. *Journal of the Generation of Human and Social Sciences,* 115–129.

Karima, B. (2016). Dyslexia and its achievement among pupils: Three class pupils as model. *Generation of Human and Social Sciences, 17–18,* 209–234.

Łodygowska, E., & Czepita, D. A. (2012). School phobia in children with dyslexia. *AnnalesAcademiaeMedicaeStetinensis, 58*(1), 66–70.

Melhem, S. M. (2000). *Find in education and science curricula psychology.* Amman: House of facilitation.

Newton, M., Thomson, M. E., & Richards, I. R. (1984). *Reading in dyslexia. A study test to accompany the Aston index.* Heinemann: LDA.

Pugh, K. R., Mencl, W. E., Jenner, A. R., Lee, J. R., Katz, L., Frost, S. J., Shaywitz, S. E., & Shaywitz, B. A. (2001). Neuroimaging studies of reading development and reading disability. *Learning Disabilities Research and Practice, 16*(4), 240–249.

Radwan, H. H. (1992). *A program to address the difficulties of learning to read and write mathematics in the fourth grade students of basic education* (Unpublished Doctoral Dissertation). Faculty of Education, Alexandria.

Rutter, M., & Yule, W. (1975). The concept of specific reading retardation. *Journal of Child Psychiatry, 16*(3), 181–197.

Saidi, A. (2009). *Introduction to dyslexia.* Amman: Dar Al - Basuri Scientific Publishing and Distribution.

Sheikh Hamoud, M. A. H., & Alammar, K. Y. (2012). *Instructional guidance for students of a class teacher.* Damascus: Faculty of Education, Damascus University, University of Damascus Publications.

Stein, J., & Glenn, C. G. (1979). An analysis of story comprehension in elementary school children. In R. O. Trudle (Ed.), *New Directions in Discarvesen Processing* (pp. 53–120). New Jersey: Ablex, Inc.

Stein, J., & Glenn, C. G. (1996). An analysis of story comprehension in elementary school children. In R. Freedle (Ed.), *Multidisciplinary perspectives in discourse comprehension* (pp. 55–110). Forwood, NJ: Ablex.

Tanner, K. (2009). Adult dyslexia and Conundrum failure. *Disability & Society, 24*(6), 785–797.

Vellutino, F. (1980). Dyslexia: Perceptual deficiency or perceptual inefficiency. In J. F. Kavanagh & R. L. Venezky (Eds.), *Orthography, reading and dyslexia* (pp. 251–270). Baltimore: University Park Press.

Vernon, M. D. (1976, July). *Heredity and environment present position of the problem.* International Congress of Psychology XXI, Paris, France.

**Beiträge zur Pädagogischen und Rehabilitationspsychologie**
**Studies in Educational and Rehabilitation Psychology**

Herausgegeben von / Edited by Evelin Witruk

Bd./Vol. 1   Evelin Witruk / David Riha / Alexandra Teichert / Norman Haase / Marcus Stueck (eds.): Learning, Adjustment and Stress Disorders. With Special Reference to Tsunami Affected Regions. 2010.

Bd./Vol. 2   Ulrike Quast: Lernermerkmale, Lernertypen, Lernverhalten. Aspekte der differentiellen Lernpsychologie für Lehrende und Lernende. 2011.

Bd./Vol. 3   Sabine Schneider: Synästhesie – Nachweis der Stabilität alphanumerischer Farbsynästhesien. 2011.

Bd./Vol. 4   Evelin Witruk / Arndt Wilcke (eds.): Historical and Cross-Cultural Aspects of Psychology. 2013.

Bd./Vol. 5   Johanna Sophie von Lieres: Tsunami in Kerala, India: Long-Term Psychological Distress, Sense of Coherence, Social Support, and Coping in a Non-Industrialized Setting. 2013.

Bd./Vol. 6   Julia Kloss: Grundschüler als Experten für Unterricht. Empirische Überprüfung der Validität von Unterrichtsbeurteilungen durch Schüler der dritten und vierten Jahrgangsstufe. 2014.

Bd./Vol. 7   Evelin Witruk / Shally Novita / Yumi Lee / Dian Sari Utami (eds.): Dyslexia and Traumatic Experiences. 2016.

Bd./Vol. 8   Evelin Witruk / Dian Sari Utami (eds.): Traumatic Experiences and Dyslexia. 2019.

www.peterlang.com

www.ingramcontent.com/pod-product-compliance
Ingram Content Group UK Ltd.
Pitfield, Milton Keynes, MK11 3LW, UK
UKHW022236230426
12048UKWH00018BA/1291